GOD'S Rx

for DEPRESSION and ANXIETY

JAMES P. GILLS, MD

SILOAM

Most CHARISMA HOUSE BOOK GROUP products are available at special quantity discounts for bulk purchase for sales promotions, premiums, fund-raising, and educational needs. For details, write Charisma House Book Group, 600 Rinehart Road, Lake Mary, Florida 32746, or telephone (407) 333-0600.

GOD'S RX FOR DEPRESSION AND ANXIETY by James P. Gills, MD
Published by Siloam
Charisma Media/Charisma House Book Group
600 Rinehart Road, Lake Mary, Florida 32746
www.charismahouse.com

Library of Congress Cataloging-in-Publication Data

Names: Gills, James P., 1934- author.
Title: God's Rx for depression and anxiety / James P. Gills.
Description: Lake Mary, Florida : Siloam, [2019] | "Portions of this book
    were originally published as Believe and Rejoice by Creation House, Lake
    Mary, FL, 2004, ISBN 1-59185-608-6, copyright " 2007.» | Includes
    bibliographical references.
Identifiers: LCCN 2019010046 (print) | LCCN 2019013529 (ebook) | ISBN
    9781629996400 (e-book) | ISBN 9781629996394 (trade paper) | ISBN
    9781629996400 (ebk.)
Subjects: LCSH: Depression, Mental--Religious aspects--Christianity. |
    Anxiety--Religious aspects--Christianity. | Spiritual
    healing--Christianity.
Classification: LCC BV4910.34 (ebook) | LCC BV4910.34 .G55 2019 (print) | DDC
    248.8/625--dc23
LC record available at https://lccn.loc.gov/2019010046

Portions of this book were originally published as *Believe and Rejoice* by Creation House, Lake Mary, FL, 2004, ISBN 1-59185-608-6, copyright © 2007.

This publication is translated in Spanish under the title *La prescripción de Dios para la depresión y la ansiedad*, copyright © 2019 by James P. Gills, MD, published by Casa Creación, a Charisma Media company. All rights reserved.

19 20 21 22 23 — 987654321
Printed in the United States of America

CONTENTS

PREFACE

THE PREMISE OF this small book is the profound dynamic of God's divine love pursuing a "heart relationship" with mankind since the beginning of time. Throughout the Scriptures this divine purpose of the loving heart of God is revealed: He created man to enjoy fellowship with Him—forever. The Shorter Catechism begins with this premise: "Man's chief end is to glorify God, and to enjoy him for ever."[1] In its essence the message of the entire Bible is that mankind was created to enjoy heart relationship with the Creator that would be characterized by His divine peace, joy, and rest—for body, mind, and spirit.

We were created with a need not just for physical rest but for divine rest—that is, harmony of spirit, soul, and body as a result of enjoying an intimate relationship with God. The Godward focus of mankind's profound friendship with God is the true source of all peace, joy, and wholeness. This supernatural well-being of believers is taught throughout the Old and New Testaments. God spoke to His people through the prophet Isaiah.

> This is the true rest [the way to true comfort and happiness] that you shall give to the weary, and, this is the [true] refreshing—yet they would not listen [to His teaching].
> —ISAIAH 28:12, AMPC

You were made to live in intimate relationship with God the Father, God the Son, and God the Holy Spirit. Then the tragedy of sin entered the human race and caused a separation between mankind and its Creator. But God designed the remedy for that separation before He ever created mankind. The Scriptures teach that Christ, our Savior, was "the Lamb slain from the foundation of the world" (Rev. 13:8). The forgiveness of sin is available to every soul who comes to Christ, the only true source of our peace, in faith. He alone can quiet the unrest of our humanity. Receiving that profound peace of God will transform the heart and mind of every person who seeks Him. He will restore you to a tranquility of a life characterized by resting in His redemption.

Redemption through Christ restores us to the heart relationships with God for which we were created. He is the remedy for depression and anxiety and other negative emotions that plague many lives to a lesser or greater degree. It is in cultivating this heart relationship that we begin to experience His profound love for us.

Perhaps we can better understand this profound spiritual reality of resting in His redemption from a conversation I had with my friend Jamie Buckingham. He had just been through a serious bout with cancer. We were walking on the beach, and I noticed that he was quieter than usual. Assuming he was feeling poorly from the treatments, I asked if he was OK. Jamie replied, "I've never been better. And my relationship with my wife is better than ever."

"But you've just been through a major health crisis," I responded. "It would be perfectly normal to be struggling right now. How can life be as good as you say?"

"Because I've come to the place where it's just Jamie and Jesus," he replied thoughtfully. "It's just Jamie and Jesus."

That is a profound life glimpse into the spiritual life of a redeemed soul who was resting in the redemption of Christ. When it's just you and God, the noisy distractions of life fade as your true priorities become crystal clear. You stop wasting time going through the motions and focus on what really matters. You live an authentic Christian life instead of "playing the part" of a Christian. Your life becomes a true reflection of the grace and loving character of our Lord. As a result, you experience a peace you've never known before, and your heart earnestly echoes the words of hymnist Horatio Spafford: "It is well with my soul."

Unfortunately that has not been the daily experience of many Christians. They either have not understood or have not availed themselves of this true rest available for every believer in Christ. Making relationship with God the priority of life and entering into intimate communion with Him is a lifelong journey. Like any human relationship, this divine relationship requires spending time with Him and learning to receive His love and return your love to Him. Sadly not all believers have made their relationship with Jesus this priority and daily focus of their lives. As a result, they try to work for Him in their own strength, and many become weary and agitated because of the complexities of life they encounter.

If you desire to experience relief from depression, anxiety, and other negative emotions that fill you with turmoil and distress, I invite you to open your heart and mind to God's rest, peace, and joy that are found only in cultivating a heart relationship of intimate communion with Him. As you journey into the unfolding truth of this wondrous mystery of God's love for you, it may seem too good to be true. That is because the love of God is unlike anything this world has to offer. Once you begin to embrace this Godward focus, you will be ruined for any lesser, temporal pleasures or loves; you will long only to taste more deeply of the divine wonder you have discovered of resting in His redemption.

—JAMES P. GILLS, MD

INTRODUCTION

MANY PEOPLE SUFFER the pain of depression and anxiety. Their struggle with these negative emotions is very real and can be devastating to their peace of mind and even their health. As Christians, we are called to do our best to reassure those struggling with negative or anxious thinking and provide them with as much comfort as possible. But for some people, this struggle goes beyond needing support. They find themselves trapped in a downward spiral of paralyzing sadness, and even common stresses of daily life overwhelm them with anxiety.

Perhaps you know someone who struggles with depression and anxiety. Maybe that someone is you. Do you find yourself unable to think clearly, sleep peacefully, or act wisely? Do even common problems of daily life overwhelm you? I encourage you to seek the help of a professional counselor or talk to your doctor. This kind of negative emotion can permeate your inner being, affecting your thoughts, attitudes, and actions. If left untreated, you can suffer emotionally, physically, and even spiritually.

This book you hold in your hands is not intended as immediate treatment for the kind of serious depression just described. It's written to help you understand that God never intended for you to have to live this way! He wants to fill your life with peace and joy! Books such as this can be a meaningful source of strength and encouragement, showing how your life can be filled with joy as you learn to rest in God's redemptive love.

To put it simply, God loves us. He is the One who saves us from sin and its devastating effects. He is our source of peace for body, mind, and spirit. That's the essence of the Christian walk. Learning to commune regularly with God as our Savior heals our soul and spirit as we receive His divine love for us. We enjoy a restful sense of His divine life within us. Oswald Chambers said that all prayer that isn't based on resting in His redemption is foolishness.[1] In other words, although you may be outwardly praying, it is of no effect if your inner man is not learning to rest in true communion with God. You are simply going through religious motions. The apostle Paul explains the effects of these faulty inner motivations in his first letter to the Corinthians.

> Though I speak with the tongues of men and of angels, but have not love, I have become sounding brass or a clanging cymbal....And though I have all faith, so that I could remove mountains, but have not love, I am nothing. And though I bestow all my goods to feed the poor, and though I give my body to be burned, *but have not love*, it profits me nothing.
> —1 CORINTHIANS 13:1–3, EMPHASIS ADDED

In the final analysis we have nothing if we do not have the love of our Creator-Redeemer, the Lord God. And His love is all we will ever need. Consider the wonder that the God who set the universe in motion also concerns Himself with the daily needs in each of our lives. And all we have to do is trust in the Savior's work on the cross, embrace His control of our lives, acknowledge His majesty and greatness, believe in His promises, and learn to live in a loving relationship with Him. In that divine relationship we will find joy and a peace that passes all human understanding. Communion with the risen Lord is to be our daily joy; this is the source of our strength in all that we do. How can we be anything but joyful when we experience a close relationship with the Creator of the universe, enjoying His peace and presence forever? For when we believe in Him and surrender ourselves to His will, our hearts are filled with a joyful spirit.

We must do all the things we do because of *having received* God's love, not in order to *obtain* God's love. The Scriptures teach that as believers, "it is God himself who has made us what we are and given us new lives from Christ Jesus; and long ages ago he planned that we should spend these lives in helping others" (Eph. 2:10, TLB). As we walk in relationship with Him, doing the work He gives us to do, there will be a natural outpouring of His divine joy in our hearts.

> These things I have spoken to you, that My joy may remain in you, and that your joy may be full.
>
> —JOHN 15:11

> As the Father loved Me, I also have loved you; abide in My love.
>
> —JOHN 15:9

We must learn to abide in His love and do everything because of God's love for us and our love for Him. Paul's prayer for the Ephesians demonstrates this principle:

> …that Christ may dwell in your hearts through faith; that you, being rooted and grounded in love, may be able to comprehend with all the saints what is the width and length and depth and height—to know the love of Christ which passes knowledge; that you may be filled with all the fullness of God.
>
> EPHESIANS 3:17–19

The Scottish minister Henry Scougal wrote that we cannot have this true joy of God until we have surrendered everything—our wants, our desires, our anger, our resentment, and our bitterness—to Him.[2] Eighteenth-century theologian and evangelist Jonathan Edwards described this profound surrender of our lives to God as the "religious affections" of grace.[3] By that he meant that we are not just surrendered; our hearts are engaged fervently in praising and worshipping God because His Word has come to us with power and we believe in Him.

The Bible teaches us that He wants our praise because we have received His salvation and we enjoy His fellowship. And then we are transformed. When we are filled with these holy "affections," life is no longer an endless search for meaning. We surrender ourselves, putting the focus of our lives on God and on worshipping Him. We are filled with the presence of God. Indeed, we must rest in His redemption, or we will never be able to worship and love Him fully. We will never have a completely joyous existence unless we worship Him with a heart of gratitude for His redemption, a heart that fervently believes in His goodness.

Believing God's promises, not just intellectually but in a faith reality of our inner being, has been the catalyst to transform the lives of millions of people and entire nations. That kind of faith reevaluates everything about us and changes our lives.

When we praise Him in gratitude for His love and redeeming power, we are filled with joy. That joy strengthens us in daily life, in our service, and in our work for God. When we do not have God's joy, the day is very long and we are less effective. When we have His joy, the day is easy.

We must examine ourselves daily and make sure we are receiving His Word and resting in His love. We must trust in God and rest in His control, letting our relationship with Him govern our lives. When we rest in His presence, we will not wrestle with Him for control. Then, when our hearts are given over to Him in faith, we are naturally filled with joy. This joy is not something we can produce ourselves. It happens only because He is at work in us and we believe in Him. He is in charge, and our relationship with Him is in order through our surrender to His loving plans for our lives.

Life is too short not to be full of joy! Life is too short to be jealous or envious of others. It is too short to be angry or resentful. It is too short to carry a grudge. It is too short to worry about material goods and be caught up in the pursuit of status or possessions. It is too short to do anything other than trust in Him, worship Him, and let His joy fill our lives.

I invite you to explore in these pages how you can rest in His redemption, believing in God, worshipping Him, and enjoying Him forever—for a joy-filled life in Him!

CHAPTER 1

GOD'S TREATMENT FOR
NEGATIVE EMOTIONS

For this reason I bow my knees to the Father of our Lord Jesus Christ, from whom the whole family in heaven and earth is named, that He would grant you, according to the riches of His glory, to be strengthened with might through His Spirit in the inner man.

—EPHESIANS 3:14–16

Humans are so much more than clumps of tissues and the results of their labor. We are not simply physical entities, as cod fish and fir trees are. We are physical, mental, emotional, and spiritual beings. Wholeness and balance at the mental and spiritual levels have been proved to affect the capacity of your body to heal physically. Additionally, as thinking, feeling products of the Creator, we have needs for mental and spiritual healing when balance has been overturned in those areas. What is required for this healing of mind and spirit? What are the ways to seek alignment in order to be healed? What is God's prescription for inner healing?

God's Word tells us that our minds need to be transformed and aligned through Christ in order for us to be the recipients of all the divine promises He has provided in our redemption (Rom. 12:1–2). It requires our full surrender to engage in this integration of the Godhead into all that we are: body, soul, and spirit. We must consecrate ourselves to Him, declaring, "Not my will, but yours be done" (Luke 22:42, NIV). This denial of self presents us to God as a holy, pleasing, and available recipient of all He is. It makes available to us the life of continual healing—health and wholeness—spiritually as well as physically. He made us to be united to Him in harmony in order for our lives to run smoothly. His main purpose for creating mankind was to draw us into fellowship with Him.

When we speak of physical health and healing, we are referring to maintaining or reacquiring balance needed for health by adhering to guidelines that the body's design dictates. Physically you align yourself with God's purpose by accepting the stewardship of your temple in which He will dwell. When we speak of balance in hearts and minds, we may think of it as realignment—that is, to prosper, you must come back into conformity, into line, with the spiritual principles and precepts by which you were created. This is the path toward healing. When that is accomplished, you may be restored to God's design and His plan.

Spiritually we must have God's Holy Spirit reigning in every part of our beings. As you yield your life to Him continually, "He will guide you into all truth" (John 16:13). He will teach you to have "the mind of Christ" (1 Cor. 2:16), showing you how to remain positive and hopeful and constantly rejoice with great feelings of thankfulness. And when you focus on eternal life rather than temporal existence, the Holy Spirit will show you how to be aligned with God and His purposes (2 Cor. 4:16–18). *Inner* healing is the healing of the mind and spirit. The body is also strengthened through the healing of your mind and spirit.

MIND AND BODY, BODY AND MIND

A merry heart does good, like medicine, but a broken spirit dries the bones.

—PROVERBS 17:22

King Solomon shows us in this proverb that he understood the requirement for health and healing; it involves wholeness of body, mind, and spirit. Intuitively we are aware that we are not divided beings into brain, body, and spirit but that each one is connected, each is a part of a singularity in its influence on each other. Those influences are more profound than we may know, however. Science is just now teasing out the details of the depth of the relationships between our brain, body, and spirit. For example, research indicates that emotional pain excites the same parts of the brain as physical pain does.

Some illnesses heal under the energies of the body's systems. Some require medical intervention, while the healing of others can be approached through diet, exercise, and lifestyle changes. And yet other illnesses can be attributed to one's mental and spiritual states. Errant emotions, fears, and anxieties can kill. Conversely realignment of your inner self can assist in your overall well-being and in your physical health.

Numerous studies have now pointed out the weight of the mind-body connection. We are being increasingly informed about the role of depression, loneliness, unhappiness, fear, and anger in the development and prolongation of diseases such as cancer, heart disease, diabetes, and asthma.[1]

Mind refers to the complete array of mental functions "related to thinking, mood, and purposive behavior. The mind is generally seen as deriving from activities in the brain but displaying emergent properties, such as consciousness."[2]

Typically we think of the mind as centered in the brain. Scientific research actually indicates that our thoughts and feelings influence the body through two primary channels: the nervous system and the circulatory system.[3] The brain, as the center of the nervous system, sends and receives electrical impulses from every part of the body. You can move a toe under the brain's instructions, and that toe also "tells" your brain, you, when it has struck something painfully. Significantly, with nerve endings in the bone marrow (the birthplace of white cells), the brain influences the mighty immune system. In addition, your brain is a gland that secretes hormones that affect the entire endocrine system.

The full depth of the mind-body connection remains somewhat of a mystery; however, every physician knows about the reality of the placebo effect. A placebo is an inert, virtually useless substance (a sugar pill, if you will) sometimes administered to a patient (normally in trials for new medications) under the pretense that it is a powerful drug that will directly improve his or her condition. Results from the administration of placebos have indeed demonstrated improvement or "healing" in statistically significant numbers of patients. Likewise, upon learning that their "medicine" was not what they believed it to be, some patients have experienced a reversion to their original sickness. There is no explanation for this outside the influence of thought and feelings on the whole person. You have heard the adage "You are what you eat." It is also true that you are what you think.

These implications are so marked that some refer to them as the "biology of belief."[4] It is in these mysterious interactions that the *body*, with its strengths and weaknesses; the *brain/mind*, with its thoughts, feelings, and consciousness; and the *spirit's* trust and communion of love with the Creator God all come together.

This complex creation that is mankind has all been planned and placed within you by design. This is not merely a combination of biology and psychology, though. As Dr. Daniel Fountain says, healing is also about faith. "Obedience to the teachings of Christ and the freeing power of the Holy Spirit can and does result in healing beyond that produced by medicine, surgery, and psychology."[5]

DEPRESSION, ANXIETY, FEAR

It has been determined by some professionals that personality is an important factor in the emergence of as well as the healing of cancer. Cancer-susceptible personalities tend to suppress toxic emotions such as anger. They also tend to suffer their burdens in life alone rather than seek comfort from others. They are also frequently unable to cope with stress. Stress is now known to suppress the immune system, and it does this more effectively in cancer-susceptible individuals, overwhelmingly so.[6]

Depression, loneliness, fear, and anxiety—these all contribute to our illnesses and play a role in the effectiveness of our healing protocols. They need not do so, however. Stress induces a stress response. The stress response involves changes in the body when an individual experiences a challenge or threat. The greater the perceived threat, the more intense and comprehensive the response. An extremely important point here is that the effects of the stress response are equivalent whether the threat is real or simply imagined.[7]

Most of us worry frequently about things that really are not exactly as they first appear to be. We imagine many things, and we make mountains out of molehills. People suffering from depression often have accompanying anxiety. They can experience panic attacks and many other physical manifestations of the overwhelming emotions they are dealing with. Worry, anxiety, and fear exaggerate our physical illnesses and impede our healing. I discuss this at greater length in another book in this series called *God's Rx for Fear and Worry*.

There is a fear that results from a basic lack of trust in Christ. Such a fear is sin. When you operate in a lack of trust in Christ, you become anxious, confused, troubled, depressed, and generally miserable. But as you grow in grace in your heart relationship with the Lord, hopefully you come to understand that the simple trusting, abiding faith you experience in His presence cannot be easily ruffled. Fear, anger, bitterness, and an underlying sense of insecurity are usually signs that somewhere along the way you have stopped relying on your faith in God and have chosen to place faith in your own abilities, independently trying to govern yourself.

In contrast, Oswald Chambers said, "*Faith* is deliberate confidence in the character of God whose ways you may not understand at the time."[8] Where and in whom our faith is established is revealed when the condition of our soul is laid bare by the onslaught of life's issues. If our faith is anchored in Him, our soul remains anchored in Him even in the thunderclouds and storms of life. If we're abiding in Him, the storms of life will not overwhelm us; if we are solely responsible for our own welfare, we'll be gripped with fear when something invades our lives that is beyond *our* capacity to resolve. Those are times when faith in God's sovereignty is a great balm to the soul!

Even tiny fears that go unchecked can build up into paralyzing trauma. To begin with, fear is understood to generate from six general categories: poverty, criticism, loss of love, illness, old age, and death. Also, fear grips a person struggling with mental disorders. This kind of fear can terrorize the mind and cripple the emotions to the point that one is bound by guilt, despair, and chronic bouts of anxiety. Instead of being productive, loss of confidence in abilities makes one ill at ease. This frame of mind can lead to being paranoid. A phobia is what results when fear and reason don't keep in touch. One more source of fear, if it is possible to separate fear into types, is physical fear. Physical fear can prevent the body's organs from functioning as God intended. It is a terrible feeling to be "physically" afraid.

God's Word is filled with promises for a life lived in peace, without fear. The psalmist said, "I will fear no evil: for thou art with me" (Ps. 23:4, KJV). David was not free from fear because there *was* no evil to fear. David's life was in danger many times while he tended his father's sheep and during the years when King Saul was trying to kill him. Yet he learned early on that God was his protector—"for thou art with me." There will always be real and genuine reasons for fear, but we can declare with David, "I will fear no evil: for thou art with me."

This doesn't mean the Christian will never suffer physical harm of any kind. No, but there is a freedom from physical fear when our confidence is grounded in God and His Word. The apostle John said, "God is love," and "Perfect love drives out fear" (1 John 4:16, 18, NIV). A relying trust in God's wisdom and love produces an abiding trust in One who has our best interests in mind. As we cultivate an intimate relationship of communion with our Lord, the Holy Spirit gives to us the mind of Christ. The apostle Paul confirmed this when he exhorted believers, "Let this mind be in you which was also in Christ Jesus" (Phil. 2:5).

Sometimes we think that Christ, who is called the Prince of Peace (Isa. 9:6), can't possibly relate to the negative feelings we suffer in our lives. However, in the Garden of Gethsemane Jesus said, "My heart is ready to break with grief" (see Matthew 26:38). Scripture says He threw Himself on the ground. This is the scene of a straining, agonizing, and struggling Jesus. The Book of Hebrews depicts the scene well: "During the days of Jesus' life on earth, he offered up prayers and petitions with fervent cries and tears to the one who could save him from death" (Heb. 5:7, NIV). He truly was "a Man of sorrows and acquainted with grief" (Isa. 53:3). Is it any wonder that He invites us into His presence? (See Matthew 11:28–29.) He wants to relieve us of fear, sorrow, and grief and fill us with His divine love that results in our peace, joy, and resting in His redemption.

We don't need to live in fear, anxiety, and depression. Our fear level is ultimately a referendum on the closeness of our friendship with God. When God says He'll never leave us or forsake us, He means it! A dear elderly patient came to the office a few years ago. After her treatment she shared her testimony.

Her Greek family first immigrated to the United States in May 1947, after the war. Though they were of Greek descent, they had been living in France and had suffered much during the war years. The family settled here in Tarpon Springs, Florida, where a large Greek community lives. She was Greek but spoke only French. It was difficult to be in an English-speaking country, living among Greek-speaking distant family members. The conditions were very difficult for her family because they had to start all over again financially. She said, "Although at first we lived in someone's garage, we didn't care that we were so poor because we were finally in a land of freedom. My sisters and I had jobs during the day, and we tried to go to language school in the evening. Times were very hard. I became sick."

All her stress affected her health. She contracted tuberculosis and was put into a sanatorium in nearby Tampa, Florida. "I was very, very lonely there. It was hard, but the Lord was very near to me. A missionary came to the sanatorium and talked about the Lord. It comforted me."

When she was finally released from the sanatorium, since she was the only unmarried daughter, it became her duty to take care of her dying mother. Her mother had been the family's tower of strength during the war, while they acclimated to a new country, and during her long illness. "When my mother died, I cried and cried and cried. I could not stop crying. After all the family members went back to their homes, I closed the curtains in my mother's home, and I sat crying day and night. My family tried to get me to go outside, but I just sat in the dark and cried. How could I go on without my mother?"

But the Lord did not leave her during this dark and lonely time. She remembered the Greek Bible that had been given to her. Though she was still learning Greek, she started to read it through from cover to cover. She said,

> The reading went very slow. As I struggled to read line after line and paragraph after paragraph, a Light began to help me understand what I was reading—it was the Holy Spirit. God's Word was like food to me. I would wake up in the middle of the night. I was reading, reading, reading, reading, all the time. I don't say that I understood all of it because it was Greek, and my childhood language was French. But I read and read and read. I read it all the way through. I have read my Bible through many times now. I do not always have the language to explain to others, but I love my Bible. I read it and read it and read it.... I read it through, then one day I opened the window shades and began to let the sunshine into the house again. The heavy depression lifted

off me. I loved my Bible. God has never failed me even in the other illnesses that I have had through the years. He is always with me in my reading of His Word. He always comes to me. I live by myself now, but I am never really alone. God is always near.

God's Word brings encouragement and divine peace and life to everyone who reads it sincerely seeking to know God. As you renew your thought life with His Word, take courage that you will be freed from depression and anxiety. God will fill you with joy and peace that passes your understanding (Phil. 4:7). In His wisdom He has provided many ways for us to be rid of negative emotions as we cultivate our intimate relationship with Him.

Medical science has discovered some of the innate healing powers God placed within our beings that, when released properly, will aid in our healing. We must remember that all healing comes from God. He is the ultimate source for the well-being of our bodies, minds, and spirits. And He will teach us to walk in wholeness with Him as we surrender our lives continually to His love.

MANAGING NEGATIVE EMOTIONS

Depression, anxiety, and fear are killers. The evidence for this conclusion is large and growing among medical professionals. Managing these negative emotions is essential to your well-being. Some people seek comfort in relationship with others, and some in the companionship of pets. To be sure, these comfort "pursuits" can have positive effects on your emotional health. Some find help as well in their involvement with a growing number of "therapies," such as art therapy (learning and practicing art). Physical exercise may be the best way to diminish unwanted stress. These are practical ways that people can help to manage negative emotions.

However, without the healing power of God working in your body, soul, and spirit, these practical therapies will not effectively eradicate the deep inner turmoil that causes negative emotional

reactions. The Scriptures teach throughout that it is impera-
tive to allow our minds to be renewed by the eternal truths the
Scriptures contain.

As we read the Word and learn how much God loves us and
desires to heal us, our faith-filled thoughts have a transforming
effect on our emotional well-being. The apostle Paul instructed
believers, "Whatsoever things are true, whatsoever things are
honest, whatsoever things are just, whatsoever things are pure,
whatsoever things are lovely, whatsoever things are of good
report...think on these things" (Phil. 4:8, KJV). The Holy Spirit
works in our hearts and minds to cleanse us of wrong thinking
and restore peace and joy to our lives.

MENTAL HEALING

It has been observed that hopelessness breeds recklessness—or,
we might say, *imbalance*. And to experience mental health, we
must walk in balance with faith and reason. Balance derives
from an understanding of and appreciation for the Creator's
wisdom. Without the awareness and appreciation, some people
seek escape from tribulation with damaging substances and
behaviors. The mental retreat into self-destructive compulsions
and addictions is frequently believed to offer answers and rest.
That is mistaken. Rather, these behaviors only complicate things
and further alienate us from the person God made us to be,
from our Creator, and from our enjoyment of knowing God and
receiving His love.

When you are faced with illness, you are presented with something that might very well be life changing in a variety of ways.
But more, through that illness you are afforded the opportunity
for personal transformation and growth. How can you make
sense of what is happening? How can you remain hopeful—how
can you live—when you are weak and fear becomes your primary
emotional response? How do you face death? How do you face
life? Who you are and how you face trouble are so important to

your overall well-being. No one can live life without facing difficult situations.

HOPE AS AN ANTIDOTE

To be able to live in hope acts as an antidote to hopelessness and depression. And it is faith that gives substance to hope: "Now faith is the *substance* of things hoped for, the evidence of things not seen" (Heb. 11:1, emphasis added). Hope is important, but hope lacks substance until it is rooted in faith in God in our hearts. I like breaking down the acronym FAITH this way: fully assured I trust Him! Hope is faith talking aloud, drowning out voices of doom and defeat. An example of one who had faith for her healing is found in Mark 5:25–28. There we read the story of the woman with the issue of blood, who said, "If only I may touch His clothes, I shall be made well." Hope gave her the tenacity to press forward in faith. The Amplified Bible, Classic Edition says, "For she kept saying, If I only touch His garments, I shall be restored to health."

Hope is birthed in an attitude of gratitude for God's love for us. A heart of thankfulness for God's love for us causes us to expect His answer for our present need joyously, even if we have to wait a little for the answer. Because we are assured of the character of God's great love for us, we can develop a habit of thankfulness toward God and others. It puts us in a frame of mind to expect to receive blessings and promises of God and to enjoy the future. Cynicism and criticism squelch hope and faith. They usually are rooted in some resentment and bitterness that haven't been dealt with yet. We can't go forward when these negative attitudes are barricading the way.

Our words are seeds that will bring a harvest. We can energize others with words of hope and plant seeds of encouragement in the lives of others and encourage our own hearts in our trying times. The Scriptures teach that "death and life are in the power of the tongue" (Prov. 18:21). Regardless of our circumstances, as we cultivate our intimate relationship with God, we are learning to trust in the loving character of God—He never fails. And we can begin to say with the psalmist, "Thy lovingkindness is better than life" (Ps. 63:3, KJV).

You can't hold back a man or woman whose hope is in the Lord from living a victorious life. To that person, God is always bigger than the giants of the Promised Land. The truths in God's Word bring hope. Saturating our souls in His Word enables us to rise above despair. Caleb and Joshua saw the giants in the land but knew that with God they could overcome (Num. 13). The prophet Jeremiah looked at the smoldering ruins of Jerusalem and responded in much the same way. He had the devastating facts, yet in the midst of his lament he reminded himself of the reliability and faithfulness of the God he served.

These patriarchs of our faith teach us valuable lessons for cultivating a heart relationship with God. No matter what life throws at us, we can learn to trust God's positive outcome as we walk in constant fellowship with Him. When Abraham was too old to receive the promise of God to him that he would have an heir, the Scriptures describe him as one "who against hope believed in hope, that he might become the father of many nations" (Rom. 4:18, KJV). It isn't human nature to hope against hope. In fact, such a response seems contrary to human sanity. But because of Abraham's faith in God's promises, his irrepressible trust in God was rewarded. God's peace passes our understanding and human reasoning (Phil. 4:6–7).

Joyous faith founded in hope cannot be explained, but it is steadfastly based on "the substance of things hoped for, the evidence of things not [yet] seen" (Heb. 11:1; cf. 1 Pet. 1:7–8). Hope breaks out of the limiting net of reasoning and moves us forward in faith and confidence in God and His Word. Hope renews our minds as we dwell in the Word of God and believe His precepts. Hebrews 6:18–19 tells us that when disappointment and confusion come, our response should be to run to the Lord, not sink into despair. God's faithfulness in times past enables us to hope again and to pass this hope along to others. Hope is "an anchor of the soul, both sure and steadfast" (v. 19).

As we receive God's Word through faith, hope rises within us. When we live it out before others as "living epistles," those who see our witness receive His living, life-giving hope just as they receive it by reading His written epistles. Their faith in Him will be enhanced when we are anchored in Him! In the times in which we live, Christians, anchored in the Rock, Christ Jesus, will be able to extend a hand of hope to those terrorized by the current events that are sure to happen before Jesus returns.

Cultivating an intimate relationship with God changes our entire perspective on life and alters its outcome as well when we discover His purposes for our lives. Spending time reading and meditating on His Word, we learn to abide in Him (John 15:4–7). In that place of abiding we enter into His profound rest and peace and enjoy who He is. It is the powerful, living Word of God, applied to our lives by the power of the Holy Spirit, that quickens the life-changing promises of God to our hearts. As you receive the love of God, being continually filled with the Spirit of God, you will find yourself resting more and more in the peace and joy of His redemption. That is the wonderful inward strength of knowing you are a child of God and enjoying your heavenly Father.

As long as you are content with a "thimbleful" of God, you will view life's challenges only from the standpoint of outward symptoms, reports of illness, bad relationship scenarios, and hopeless circumstances. Your soul will be troubled by a myriad of negative emotions as a result. In contrast, hope in God and His Word will transform you into a man or woman of faith. The Word of God comes alive in you when you call upon the Holy Spirit of God to awaken your spirit and soul to who God is. Let the words of Jeremiah remind you of the omnipotence of God: "There is nothing too hard for thee" (Jer. 32:17, KJV).

DISCUSSION ❧ QUESTIONS

List the negative emotions you've been dealing with.

....

....

....

What physical symptoms are you experiencing that might be connected to the negative emotions in your life?

....

....

....

What will you do to deepen and strengthen your heart relationship with Christ and discover the peace and joy He promises all believers?

....

....

....

Write a scripture that gives you hope.

....

....

....

CHAPTER 2

A HEART OF FAITH,
A LIFE OF JOY

*Glory in his holy name; let the hearts of
those who seek the LORD rejoice.*
—1 CHRONICLES 16:10, NIV

HINK ABOUT THE word *joy*. What image comes to mind? Angels in the heavens announcing the birth of Christ? A child full of laughter and happiness? Beethoven's beautiful ninth symphony? Nineteenth-century preacher C. H. Spurgeon said, "Joy is peace dancing."[1] What a wonderful image!

God wants us to have a life filled with more joy than we can ever imagine. It doesn't happen by accident, but it does surprise us. Author C. S. Lewis wrote that we find joy only when we are looking for something else.[2] And that something else is God. It is a one-two punch: we seek God, really believing in Him, and we find joy. Lewis said it more eloquently: joy is the response or result of the felt sense of God's love in our soul. Again, it is the inner disposition of profound enjoyment of God's presence in our lives that fills our hearts with His peace and joy.

It is a journey we undertake when we turn our lives over to God. When we truly believe in God, we surrender every worry, every concern, and every aspect of our lives to Him. We are concerned only about living in God's presence and believing in His promises. The apostle Paul described three critical elements in this journey to a joy-filled life: relinquishment, faith, and grace.

> I have been crucified with Christ and I no longer live, but Christ lives in me. The life I now live in the body, I live by faith in the Son of God, who loved me and gave himself for me.
>
> —GALATIANS 2:20, NIV

Sometimes we are reluctant to talk about joy and God. We tend to associate joy with comfort, ease, and luxury. But joy is a much deeper and richer experience than those words describe. The joy God gives is the natural outpouring of our hearts as God's presence becomes the central pillar of our lives. When we have a personal relationship with Him, we cannot help but be filled with heavenly, glorious joy that is expressed in a deep desire to worship and adore God. Having His divine presence in our lives is the ultimate joy and satisfaction to the human heart.

How do we come to know God in that kind of personal relationship? First we have to acknowledge God as our Creator. Then we have to really believe in Christ as God's Son, who became our Savior. We have to love Him and trust Him enough to embrace His rule over our lives. There is an old-fashioned word that is used to describe this process of learning to trust: relinquishment. The dictionary says that *relinquish* means "to let go of; give up; surrender."[3] When we are passengers in a car, we have to relinquish control to the person behind the wheel, or we take the terrible role of backseat drivers.

Relinquishment is a combination of surrendering your will and entrusting yourself to God. *Surrender* is a parallel response to God with repentance; *entrusting* your life to Him is a way of expressing faith. The apostle Paul summarized his teaching of the whole counsel of God in these words: "repentance toward God and faith toward our Lord Jesus Christ" (Acts 20:21).

For Christians, *relinquishment to God* means surrendering the plans for our lives, giving up our wants and desires, cares and worries, abandoning our selfish nature, receiving God's love, trusting His provision, and experiencing His filling with the Holy Spirit. Our faith enables us to leave behind all the cares and concerns of this world. We can call it "abandoned faith" because we are abandoning the values and goals of the world for a life of faith in God. We are filled with trust in God, and we relinquish control to Him. In that place of surrender to His love, we discover that we are filled with His abundant, glorious joy. In that place we find true rest in His redemption and begin to live an authentic Christian life that reflects the graces and character of our Savior.

The experience of John Wesley, the great evangelist and founder of the Methodist movement, shows how abandoned faith can change a life. By the time he was thirty-five Wesley knew a lot about Christ. He had graduated from Oxford University and resolved to become a priest in the Church of England. He was ordained a priest in 1728. He and his brother, Charles, helped start the Holy Club at Oxford. He read one hundred spiritual books a year for a dozen years. He even traveled to Georgia on a mission trip. But he knew there was something missing. On his mission trip he met some Moravian immigrants who had the spiritual peace he realized he was lacking. Because his work in America was not very effective, he decided to return to England.

Back in London, Wesley met Peter Böhler, another Moravian, who convinced him that what he needed was simple: he needed faith, not just knowledge about God. During a meeting on Aldersgate Street in 1738, Wesley was transformed. As he heard Martin Luther's preface to the *Commentary on Romans* being read, he was truly elated. He realized the promises of God are true! He wrote, "I felt my heart strangely warmed. I felt I did trust in Christ, Christ alone, for salvation."[4] He felt a quickening that comes from truly experiencing God's grace and presence. And he was filled with God's complete and perfect joy. From that point on Wesley was a changed man. He preached with a spiritual fire and fervor that was fed by his faith. And he was filled with a glorious joy that affected him the rest of his life because his life was relinquished to God and he believed in His promises.

We can have the same kind of life filled with abandoned faith and joy. It's a faith and a joy that come from inner harmony, the true rest Christ came to give every believer. We experience a victorious counteraction to our internal struggles. And we learn the futility of complaining about trouble and worrying about trying to control the future. When we believe in God's promises and trust Him to be in control of our lives, joy is the glorious result. We do not have joy; it has us. Our joy in God is based on His delight in us. (See Psalm 149:4.)

What an offer! If we quit worrying about our own lives and trust God to do the driving, we will find our lives full of blessings and riches beyond our wildest dreams. We cannot even begin to know all the blessings we will receive from His loving hand.

Indeed, if we consider the unblushing promises of reward and the staggering nature of the rewards promised in the Gospels, it would seem that our Lord finds that our desires are not too strong but too weak. We are half-hearted creatures, fooling about with drink and sex and ambition when infinite joy is offered us, like an ignorant child who wants to go on making mud pies in a slum because he cannot imagine what is meant by the offer of a holiday at the sea. We are far too easily pleased.[5]

The purpose for writing this book is to encourage and inspire every reader to experience a deeper reality of God's love for him or her, to help the reader develop a Godward focus in order to realize the inner peace and joy God gives, regardless of the outward circumstances of our lives that seem difficult. In this study, through our reading, exploration of the Word, and prayer together, that is what we will find—the infinite, glorious joy that results from believing in God.

Dear Lord Jesus, bless us as we discover Your truths and learn to love You as You love us.

DISCUSSION 🌿 QUESTIONS

What does *joy* mean to you?

....

....

....

....

Describe a person or event in your life that brought you joy. Did that joy last, or was it temporary?

....

....

....

....

Have you ever experienced the kind of joy that Wesley experienced, one that comes from renewed faith and a deeper sense of God's presence?

....

....

....

....

CHAPTER 3

THE JOY OF
SALVATION

*The Lord your God is with you, the Mighty Warrior who
saves. He will take great delight in you; in his love he will
no longer rebuke you, but will rejoice over you with singing.*
—ZEPHANIAH 3:17, NIV

OD'S Rx FOR living a life of joy, free from depression
and anxiety, is available only in our pursuit of the inner
strength we find in cultivating an intimate relationship
with God. Perhaps everyone has at some time struggled to
find joy, thinking that when he achieves the "right" thing
in work, play, or relationships, he will know the joy that seems
so elusive. Yet when we approach life in this way, we create such
hectic days full of activities and accomplishments that we think
a filled life is the same as a fulfilled life. We seek recreations on
a basketball court, in a gym, or on a bicycle that engage us for
the moment but are not lasting. Or we search for that "special
someone," only to discover that our problem is not in finding the
right person but in not being the right people ourselves.

C. S. Lewis said that each of us has this kind of deep longing
that we search to fill. He calls it *sehnsucht*, or a longing for joy.[1]

Because we are human, we try to fill it with earthly things. The divine inner quality of joy eludes us as we search instead for happiness in our personal pursuits. We say, "If I can just get my education finished and get started in my career, then things will go well, and I will be happy." But when we achieve that goal, we are not happy. So we say, "If I can just get established in my business and be successful, then things will go well, and I will be happy." But it doesn't happen. Then we think, "Well, if I can just find the right spouse and have good children, then things will go well, and I will be happy." But that still doesn't satisfy us. So then we say, "If I can just get the kids through school, then I can settle down and rest." But still we are missing the point.

There are simply no magic plateaus where our lives level off and we think we have achieved happiness. Personal achievements, success at work or on the athletic field, and relationships cannot give us lasting joy. We can have all those things and still feel this empty longing to which C. S. Lewis referred. At some point in our lives we have to realize that what we seek isn't within our power to achieve; we lack the inner resources to fill this void. When we finally see how weak we are, how limited our powers are, we can be eaten up with depression, frustration, anger, anxiety, and loneliness.

Then God speaks to us. And for the first time we truly begin to see the power and majesty of the almighty God. We see ourselves as poor, needy sinners who need the grace of the Lord Jesus and His cross. We turn to God because we realize we have nowhere else to go. The apostle Paul explains salvation in clear terms.

> Because of his kindness, you have been saved through trusting Christ. And even trusting is not of yourselves; it too is a gift from God. Salvation is not a reward for the good we have done, so none of us can take any credit for it. It is God himself who has made us what we are and

> given us new lives from Christ Jesus; and long ages ago he
> planned that we should spend these lives in helping others.
> —EPHESIANS 2:8–10, TLB

Paul tells us in these verses first that it is only God's grace that can save us. Salvation is His gift to us. And second that God has a plan for our lives—to spend these lives in helping others. How wonderful is this thought that God has a special purpose for us to fulfill in the earth. As we walk with Christ, cultivating relationship with Him, He reveals His plan for our lives, vocationally, in our relationships, and in every area of our lives. And He gives us His grace to fulfill His will and enjoy the ultimate fulfillment in life that He gives as we rest in His redemption.

Grace is a biblical word that can be the greatest word you hear or the word you let pass by without interest. If you are self-sufficient, proud, and self-righteous, you do not think you need God's grace. On the other hand, if you feel humbled or even humiliated because of your failings—your sins—you may hesitate to believe that there is a possibility of redeeming grace for your life.

The apostle Paul was ashamed of how he tried to exterminate Christians before his conversion, but the grace of God even changed Paul's heart and filled him with the joy of forgiveness. He described the grace of God working in his life.

> For I am the least of the apostles, who am not worthy to
> be called an apostle, because I persecuted the church of
> God. But by the grace of God I am what I am.
> —1 CORINTHIANS 15:9–10

Paul called himself the chief of sinners (1 Tim. 1:15) and felt he was "less than the least of all the saints" (Eph. 3:8). He was amazed that God would graciously forgive all his sins because of what Jesus did on the cross to save him. Yet he did believe the good news of the gospel and spent his life spreading that good news to others.

The Philippian jailer probably felt there was little hope for him as an enemy of God's apostles, roughly throwing them into the inner prison and putting them into stocks. Yet Paul boldly proclaimed to him, "Believe on the Lord Jesus Christ, and you will be saved" (Acts 16:31). This same promise is true for you and me. Let us cast ourselves upon God's mercy and grace. We will find that God delights to show mercy (Mic. 7:18) and will forgive us and make us His own children. God says it! Let's believe it!

How gracious and sweet is God's invitation. He throws His arms around us when we fall at His feet and say, "Lord, we are poor, worthless sinners. Please, in Your everlasting mercy and grace, accept us, take us, let us be Yours. Be our Redeemer, Savior, and Friend, for we trust and believe in You, and we love You."

May God flood our souls with the divine joy of God's true salvation. May we begin to see the infinite majesty of God and the eternal love He desires to give us. And let us ever be grateful to Him that He has given us hope and joy in believing!

> Then my soul will rejoice in the LORD and delight in his salvation.
>
> —PSALM 35:9, NIV

Joy is the expression of a heart that is changed by embracing an intimate relationship with God. He fills us with His love that takes our breath away. His love resounds within our hearts like an infinite host of angels singing glory to God. It is the greatest music or words we can ever imagine, and still more. This great joy puts everything else out of our heads and our hearts. In turning from earthly things, we find God. And by putting our faith in Him, we are filled with abundant joy. Gone are the negative emotions of depression and anxiety, the hopelessness, the sense of futility in life that once plagued our hearts and minds. Instead, we are bathed in His overwhelming love, peace, and joy that fill our hearts and minds and put a smile on our lips.

If you have not received Jesus as your personal Savior and heavenly Friend, pray with me.

Lord, I realize how far short I have fallen. I know I'm not worthy of Your love. But through the miracle of Your grace, forgive me and make me Your child. Help me turn to You and love You. Show me how to live and love and be like You.

DISCUSSION ❦ QUESTIONS

Reflect for a moment on God's incredible gift of mercy and grace through salvation. Describe how it makes you feel.

....

....

....

....

....

How has knowing God changed you and the course of your life?

....

....

....

....

Write a scripture that reminds you of the miracle of your salvation.

....

....

....

....

....

CHAPTER 4

LEARNING
TO REST

WE CANNOT HAVE a life filled with joy without God's divine love. When two people fall in love, a natural joy springs up and fills them with an unconditional love for each other. That is the impact the divine joy we receive through our salvation in Christ has on our hearts; He is someone who loves us far more than anyone else ever could. This new heart relationship is filled with a wonderful sense of God's love and joy. The Bible refers to God's love for us as delight. "For the LORD takes delight in his people" (Ps. 149:4, NIV). God takes pleasure in us, and we rejoice in that and take pleasure in Him. We are joyful in our King. Love is essential to a life of faith and joy. God's Word tells us just how important love is.

> Love the LORD your God with all your heart, with all your soul, and with all your strength.
> —DEUTERONOMY 6:5

Jesus referred to this commandment as the most important of God's commandments (Matt. 22:37–38). For any of us love demonstrates the visible reality of a life that is surrendered in faith to

God. Without love our actions and words are meaningless. As I mentioned in the introduction, 1 Corinthians 13 says that we can have the gift of prophecy, understand all mysteries and knowledge, have faith to move mountains, give all our goods to the poor, and have our body burned. And we can have all sorts of abilities to speak. But unless we are resting in the redemption and love of Christ, all these spiritual gifts and abilities do us no good. Churches or people who do not embrace love as Christ desires we experience in Him give Christianity a cold appearance. They have not embraced the Godward focus that is intimate relationship with God, who is love (1 John 4:8).

As we tell God He is wonderful, we are in love with Him. It is like a marriage. As a man tells his wife that she is wonderful, he is in love with her. Look at couples who struggle in their marriages. Insecurities, pride, hostility, and many other forms of selfishness keep them from becoming close and surrendering to one another.

We have the same problems in our relationship with Christ. We all have anxieties, frustrations, and doubts. But God commands us to turn them over to Him. He calls us to love Him and be in communion with Him. A heart filled with love has less room for selfishness. As we love God more and more, we can surrender more and more of ourselves—and the more we can rest in our redemption.

We need to be able to look up to Jesus by faith and say, "Jesus, You're wonderful. I love You, and I am Your child—Your spiritual child, Your child for eternity."

SWEET SURRENDER

If we are really going to be committed to God, we have to be committed to living a life that honors Him. We have to be able to say, "Lord, You're in charge now. I put all my faith in You. You lead; I'll follow." We must give up our worldly agendas and desires and trust His control of our lives. Then we find happiness, not by worldly standards—achieving our goals of success, fame, money, or power. We find true joy filling our hearts through the outpouring of the love of our Creator and Redeemer into our hearts. (See Romans 5:5.) Then we pour out our love to Him and toward others.

Think about it again like a marriage. A man loves his wife. He wants what she wants; he sacrifices for her. He surrenders himself to the joy of knowing, caring for, and appreciating her. One verse that describes a healthy marriage repeats what Adam said of Eve: "This is now bone of my bones and flesh of my flesh" (Gen. 2:23). That picture of intimacy helps all of us remember that in marriage we can't really become one person, one partnership living in harmony, until we surrender ourselves to each other in love.

And just as any of us surrender to our spouses, so we must surrender ourselves to our God. Surrendering to God, we become one with Him spiritually in heart and joyfully in reality! We love and trust God so completely that we can surrender our lives to Him. Love gives us the strength and trust to turn everything over to Him. Paul gives us a road map in Galatians 2:20 for this journey. It involves surrender, faith, and grace. Let's look again at his testimony.

> I have been crucified with Christ and I no longer live, but Christ lives in me.
>
> —GALATIANS 2:20, NIV

What Paul says so beautifully is that we cannot live in Christ until we are ready to die to self—our own wants, desires, and egos. Jesus also spoke of it.

> Then He said to them all, "If anyone desires to come after Me, let him deny himself, and take up his cross daily, and follow Me. For whoever desires to save his life will lose it, but whoever loses his life for My sake will save it."
>
> —LUKE 9:23–24

I tell you, unless a kernel of wheat falls to the ground and dies, it remains only a single seed. But if it dies, it produces many seeds. Anyone who loves their life will lose it, while anyone who hates their life in this world will keep it for eternal life.

—JOHN 12:24–25, NIV

Paul also writes about it.

I face death every day—yes, just as surely as I boast about you in Christ Jesus our Lord.

—1 CORINTHIANS 15:31, NIV

We always carry around in our body the death of Jesus, so that the life of Jesus may also be revealed in our body.

—2 CORINTHIANS 4:10, NIV

We must die to our selfishness before we can truly appreciate God. We must give up our egos and all that goes with them—pride and the desire for control, worldly status, and success. This is what it means to be born again of the Spirit. And we must follow the scriptural command to "present your bodies a living sacrifice, holy, acceptable to God, which is your reasonable service" (Rom. 12:1). The world and all its lures, temptations, and struggles must no longer have a controlling grip on our lives. We belong to God, and He lives in us. The Bible warns us about the wrong involvement in worldly affairs.

Do you not know that friendship with the world is enmity with God? Whoever therefore wants to be a friend of the world makes himself an enemy of God.

—JAMES 4:4

Everybody knows you must take risks to be successful by earthly standards. What we risk in order to make anything of our lives spiritually is even greater. We have to risk worldly success, risk losing our feeling of independence, and risk giving up control of our lives. But what we gain is so great that the risks pale in comparison. Charles Swindoll asked, "Are you willing to risk as much to make a difference as you are willing to risk to make a dollar?"[1] To truly rest in His redemption, we have to risk it all, as the apostle Paul wrote.

> I consider everything a loss because of the surpassing worth of knowing Christ Jesus my Lord, for whose sake I have lost all things. I consider them garbage, that I may gain Christ and be found in him.
> —PHILIPPIANS 3:8–9, NIV

> *Dear heavenly Father, I believe You love me and sent Your Son to save me. Help me to lovingly surrender every area and aspect of my life to You, that I may honor and glorify Your name above all others.*

FAITH: THE SIXTH SENSE

> The life which I now live in the flesh I live by faith in the Son of God.
> —GALATIANS 2:20

Faith is really a sixth sense. The first five senses—touch, taste, smell, hearing, and sight—are in carnal man. The sixth sense is in the spiritual man. The natural unregenerate man cannot appreciate faith any more than the sense of hearing appreciates the sense of smell. But the sixth sense is absolutely essential if we are going to live complete lives full of joy. In seeking God, faith is given to us as we hear His Word.

> Consequently, faith comes from hearing the message, and the message is heard through the word about Christ.
> —ROMANS 10:17, NIV

Let's look at the word *faith*. Hebrews 11:6 tells us to diligently seek God, emphasizing that faith isn't simply an intellectual exercise. Instead, faith is our conviction, and by faith we rest in Him, abide in Him, and draw strength from Him.

Great athletes must forget about everything else so they can train and play wholeheartedly. If they worry about getting injured or worry about how other athletes are doing, they cannot perform well. They cannot focus. That is a picture of the essence of abandoned faith to the Lord: giving everything wholeheartedly to Him—every worry, concern, desire, and goal.

It is a faith that is not just in our minds; it is a faith that believes all the promises of God. We must have a total abandonment spiritually, totally trusting in the Lord. The joy in our hearts that comes from abandonment to Him keeps us from worrying about the cares of the day, the politics of the day, and the cynicism of the day. His joy lets us be concerned only about being totally abandoned and surrendered to the Lord.

The battle we have with our fallen inclinations is won in our hearts with God when we believe in Him. Then we step into a life of faith. And when we fully believe in God and His promises, we have an abandoned faith that focuses on God and forgets the world.

Look at the example of Robert Morrison. He was one of the first missionaries to China in the early 1800s. As he was sailing to China, the captain of the ship asked, rather sarcastically, "So, Mr. Morrison, you expect to make an impression on the great empire of China, do you?" Morrison replied, "No, I expect God will."[2] What a shining example of believing God's promises! Morrison served twenty-seven years in China, and he is considered the father of Protestant mission work there.

It doesn't take a great mind or years of education to have such abandoned faith. As the old hymn says, "Trust and obey, for there's no other way."[3] All each of us needs to do is trust in God and believe in His promises.

However, we can believe in either the right things or the wrong things. What are some deceptions that we should not start believing? "Life should be fair." "My unhappiness is because of someone else." "My good is determined by what I can do." "Our marriage requires too much work; we must not be right for each other." We start believing there are certain things we can do or things we can own that will solve our problems and fill our longings. But when we start seeking things that are not focused on God, we no longer have abandoned faith in Him. Instead, we start to abandon our faith in His promises to walk independently in what we think we can achieve ourselves.

We need not be deceived by the difficult times in our lives. God promises to help us through them. All we need to believe is that His grace is sufficient and all our blessings come because we believe in Him. And as we bow before Him in abandoned faith and gratitude for His love and His redemption, we will know His love in a deeper way than before. And in that place of abandonment to His love, no negative emotion such as depression or anxiety will survive.

> *Dear Father, thank You for being so good to me. May my faith and trust in You grow daily.*

COMMUNION AND CONVERSATION

When we love God, we want to be in His presence, and we want to talk with Him and share ourselves with Him. Prayer is one way we can be in constant communion with Him. In prayer we make the nearest approach to God. It opens the inward thoughts of both God and man, and true intimacy is found. In true sincerity we must open our hearts to God in prayer—sometimes with thoughtful, eloquent prayers; sometimes with words that cannot be uttered; sometimes with thoughts that cannot be translated. And then our hearts and our total beings are surrendered in intimacy to Him.

Fervent and hearty prayer is necessary. All-day-long prayers are sometimes necessary as we seek to know the mind of God for our lives. This life of prayer should be a state of meditation on the glory of God. We must have this kind of personal, vital relationship with Him. Otherwise Christianity becomes a joyless burden, and at the end of our lives we will regret that we didn't pray, because we didn't surrender ourselves and rest in His redemption.

This intimacy through prayer leads to fulfillment of joy because prayer is the nerve center of our vital fellowship with Jesus. It brings us a life filled with deep, abiding joy. As 1 John 1:3–4 says, "Our fellowship is with the Father and with his Son, Jesus Christ. We write this to make our joy complete" (NIV).

We measure fluids by gallons. Some measure a dog's value by its loyalty to its master. Others may measure a dog's value by how much an owner is willing to pay a veterinarian for the dog's health care. Scripture teaches us to measure ourselves spiritually by the quality of our prayer lives. We can measure the quality of our prayer lives by asking ourselves how genuinely we praise God, how intently we draw near to God, and how effectively we are being transformed into His image. The apostle Paul expressed the transformative power of prayer and waiting on God in this way: "But we all, with open face beholding as in a glass the glory of the Lord, are changed into the same image from glory to glory, even as by the Spirit of the Lord" (2 Cor. 3:18, KJV).

We become like what we love and honor. One way to show our love and honor for God is through prayer. That life of communion with God gives us all we need—peace and joy—for today and for eternity.

Father, let me love You and in love surrender to You,
to Your grace, to Your will, with the help of the Holy
Spirit filling me with Your presence.

THE HELP OF THE HOLY SPIRIT

No matter how much we try to "will" ourselves to surrender everything to God, it is something we cannot do alone. In marriage our spouses help us. To truly rest in His redemption, we need the Holy Spirit working in us. C. H. Spurgeon said, "There are times when I've been a half-inch from heaven and you've been a half-inch from heaven."[4] The Holy Spirit makes that difference as we focus on Him and wait for His Spirit and His closeness. His *shekinah* glory, the manifested glory of God, fills us, displacing the rest of the world. Then we are able to empty ourselves of the world, and He fills us with Himself.

Moses gives us a vivid example of a life filled with this kind of glory in Exodus 34:29–35. He had a physical reflection of the *shekinah* glory because he was so close to the Lord that he radiated with the glory of the Lord. And those around him would be alarmed by the glorious radiance of the Lord's presence seen in the face of Moses. The *shekinah* glory is not something just for Old Testament prophets, however. It is for all of us today as we seek His presence.

> For God, who said, "Let light shine out of darkness," made his light shine in our hearts to give us the light of the knowledge of God's glory displayed in the face of Christ.
>
> —2 CORINTHIANS 4:6, NIV

And that glory comes through the work of the Holy Spirit. John 1:4 says that in Jesus "was life, and that life was the light of all mankind" (NIV). So Jesus, as the Light of life, through the Holy Spirit, gives light upon the holy things of God. We need to commune with God, Jesus, and the Holy Spirit, each distinctly and all wrapped together to give us the joy that results from being present with Him. *Shekinah* glory comes only when we have a spirit of repentance and faith that loves Him, delights in Him, and worships Him. Then His *shekinah* glory is present within us, radiating into us and out into the world.

Have you ever known someone who had an aura of radiance? He might not have said anything holy, but his life was filled with the presence of the Holy Spirit. He was full of the love of God and was completely surrendered to Him, letting Him direct his life. This spirit of joy, peace, and thanksgiving is truly a wonderful sight.

The Israelites discovered that truth in the Old Testament. When they came out of their captivity in Babylon, they had nothing but the Word of God. When they heard it, they understood it and went their way, rejoicing. They understood that though they had no material goods, they should not grieve and mourn. Being in God's presence is joyous and completely fulfilling.

The radiance of the Holy Spirit lets everyone see that we are truly His. It enables us to reflect Christ and His love. We can be like the people with that holy aura. We don't need to speak. We just let the light of Christ shine in our lives. The Holy Spirit can permeate the lives of each of us so we will think differently, act differently, and live differently.

The Israelites celebrated the Feast of Tabernacles, a feast of thanksgiving that honors God as the host and the Israelites as the guests. In the same way, we daily should come to the Word of God and rejoice in His presence because we have faith in Him and in His Spirit. We can describe the smile of God upon our hearts that allows us to speak His Word as a divine unction or fervor. This is God's holiness speaking through us. Jesus' disciples demonstrated this divine unction.

> And the disciples were filled with joy and with the Holy Spirit.
>
> —ACTS 13:52

The disciples were infused with this joy and the Holy Spirit because their hearts were joined to God and filled with His presence. A few verses earlier we learn that when the Gentiles heard the good news of the gospel, they rejoiced, praising and honoring the Word of God. (See Acts 13:48.) They were filled with joy because it came from the praise that the Holy Spirit stirred up within them, and that praise changed their inner beings and gave them true joy. When the Holy Spirit gives us His glory, we need to enjoy it and cherish it and tell Him how wonderful He is to give it to us.

Tony Evans describes the importance of the Holy Spirit in the believer's life in a surprising manner.[5] His analogy is "jumper cables" from Jesus to us. Can you imagine having jumper cables to use in the morning to get your mind turned on right? Jumper cables for feeling the promises of God are true for your whole being? They are jumper cables that really make us feel that Jesus is within us by the power of the Holy Spirit. Evans' analogy of the Holy Spirit is just one of the many descriptions of how God works in us when we give ourselves to be abandoned to Him and seek the Holy Spirit to work through us. All of this is to one end: to glorify Him and to live with Him in love, enjoying Him and glorifying Him forever.

FINDING FELICITY

Felicity was a servant-saint who lived around the year AD 200. She was executed because she refused to renounce her belief in God. Even when she was put in an arena with a wild bull, she did not deny Christ but died praising Him. Hers is a story of a girl who desired God above all things. Felicity's devotion to Christ teaches us that it is possible to have God's ultimate joy if we truly believe and trust in Him, regardless of our circumstances. That attitude can be called *felicity*—God's tranquility personified. Felicity, the saint, had that divine presence within her. We should seek the same. Her faith in God and love for Him set a powerful example for us today.

When we come to God in repentance and faith, we rest in the peace that He will be Jehovah Jireh—the great Provider of all. (See Genesis 22:14.) We have satisfaction, peace, and joy in God. This is evidence that we are in right standing with God and that we are subduing our sinful nature. Then the things of the world will be put in the proper perspective, and we will enjoy them more because we are aligned with Him.

The blessedness we receive from God is filling and satisfying. The satisfactions we try to get from the world—material goods, admiration and respect from others, and sensual pleasures—in the long run leave us with the greatest emptiness. We think they will satisfy us, but they never live up to our expectations. The emptiness that follows is overwhelming and leads to the greatest despair, even when we have everything we want. When football players in the NFL win that championship ring—something they have sought their whole careers—there can be the greatest sense of emptiness in possessing that ring if that is all they have. Without relationship with God, even the greatest achievements in life fail to satisfy our deepest longings for fulfillment. True felicity and satisfaction are not present in the world; they are present only in knowing Christ.

We become like God when we receive His love and in return love Him with all our hearts. What is it that rules in our hearts? Is it love to God? God's Word tells us what love to God is like. When we love God, we will seek to do what God's Word says. (See 1 John 5:3.) It is important that we feel God's love for us. When we are dull of heart, we need to seek Him to rekindle in our hearts that sense of His great love for us.

Richard Baxter, a seventeenth-century theologian, noted that love, desire, hope, and courage lead us to a joy in God. He said these emotions, these affections or influences over the heart, flow from our innermost being as we praise God for the excellence of Christ. Then we turn away and find that external joys mean nothing without Christ in them. That is a dangerous place to live where depression and anxiety lurk.

We call it "enlarging the neck" when we embrace the inner disposition of giving God our affections because these affections basically make an opening between the head and heart. Everything we think about must be contemplated in godly ways, and those things become part of our hearts and permeate our whole bodies. While it's important to think about these things, it is also important to have lively affections for them. We cannot only make logic within our heads; we must praise with our hearts.

A person's heart relationship with God is the source of her joy. Everything we do in living our lives in communion with God must promote that joy. It is necessary for the heart to elevate the soul in what Baxter called "heavenly contemplations."[6] We must love and be loved. Then we feel this felicity, this afterglow, this all-desiring affection of being close to God.

Felicity is a descriptive way of referring to the influence of the Holy Spirit in our lives. He helps us develop the fruit of the Spirit in our lives (Gal. 5:22–23), including joy and contentment. Yet felicity is not always consistent in our affections because we are not always totally committed to the Lord. For heaven knows that all of us have let our thoughts and our actions become sinful and as a result have felt the eclipse of God's felicity and tranquility. There are times when we are very full of everything in life that is not of felicity. We are filled with the things of the world, and we are taken away from our fellowship with the Lord. Happily, when we remember the times of the greatest felicity we once experienced, it breaks our hearts and brings us back to seek the Lord again. We are restored to His presence through repentance and no longer travel the road that leads to further deceit and hurt.

So often we have wandered along and contented ourselves with vain shadows and false imaginations of piety and religion, not truly believing in His promises. The affections that lead to felicity are stirred by divine impressions and touched by our faith in Him. When we see a fellow brother or sister in Christ, and he has an abundance of joy and happiness, we are seeing the Holy Spirit's overflow of joy in his life. This is the blessing we must seek with our whole heart. Let each of us pray.

> Lord, help me open my eyes and see that my whole purpose is to love You and enjoy You forever in a state of joy and contentment in the Holy Spirit.

DISCUSSION ✤ QUESTIONS

Can you think of an example in your life of the connection between joy, love, and surrender? Describe it.

_____

_____

_____

How does your prayer life affect your relationship with God? Do you view it as a two-way conversation between you and the Lord?

_____

_____

_____

Are there things you need to reprioritize to make sure your prayer time with God comes first?

_____

_____

_____

How does the Holy Spirit help you in this process?

_____

_____

_____

CHAPTER 5

TRAITS OF A
RESTED LIFE

ARL PALMER, IN discussing C. S. Lewis' *Screwtape Letters*, described joy as a "meaningful acceleration, a rhythm with the character of God."[1] We don't sit still. We physically and mentally become more and more involved in the righteous, loving character of God because we are surrendered to Him. Let's go back to Galatians 2:20. It says, "I no longer live, but Christ lives in me" (NIV). This means we want what God wants. We become more and more like Him. And as we are filled with His love, negative emotions are expelled from our psyches. Our hearts are at rest as we find our inner strength in God.

Have you ever been around a couple who have been married a long time? Their marriage has transformed them. They have become like each other. In fact, sometimes they finish each other's sentences because they are of one mind and heart. There is a harmony between them. Their love for each other fills them with joy, peace, gentleness, and goodness. And that attitude carries over into their relationships with other people. Their loving relationship has truly united them.

A heart that is resting in redemption, a "rested heart," is not one that is proud of its commitment, nor does it feel self-righteous. No, it is one that realizes, "I am nothing; Jesus is everything. I can do nothing. I need Him for everything." A resting heart is a heart that is broken and emptied of the love of self. It is filled with humble gratitude because of the realization that the Son of God would love and pity us when we were still sinners and then fill us with His gracious presence when we turn our hearts toward Him.

When we rest in God's redemption, truly surrendering our lives to Him, we receive divine life through our Lord and Savior. Our surrendered hearts find joy in the Lord, and our lives are filled with the same spiritual qualities as that married couple—love, joy, peace, patience, kindness, goodness, faithfulness, gentleness, and self-control. (See Galatians 5:22–23.) This fruit of the Holy Spirit changes us, and our relationships with others change as a result.

As we stand close to God, His image is stamped on us. We are transformed. It cannot be any other way. It is inevitable that we are changed because the Holy Spirit lives in us. The apostle Paul instructed us to live and walk in that relationship with God, renouncing the former attachments to the ways of the world.

> Do not be conformed to this world, but be transformed
> by the renewing of your mind, that you may prove what
> is that good and acceptable and perfect will of God.
> —ROMANS 12:2

Our being must be transformed from the inside out. Our old thought processes must be taken captive as we are renewed by His Word and in prayer and worship—through the enablement and encouragement of the Holy Spirit. Our lives are changed as we cultivate an intimate relationship with our Savior, communing with Him continually through prayer and the study of His Word. Let's look at some of the dramatic changes that occur as we give our hearts and minds to God.

THE ETERNAL VIEW

A lot of people are nearsighted. They see only the things that are up close. All of us can be nearsighted spiritually, seeing only the things that are up close in ourselves and in those around us. We can fail to see the overall view. James 4:14 describes this nearsightedness: "Why, you do not even know what will happen tomorrow. What is your life? You are a mist that appears for a little while and then vanishes" (NIV).

Our perspective of life is small when we don't rest in God's love, fully surrendered to Him with the help of the Holy Spirit. When we are selfish and caught up in our own daily dramas, we cannot truly see. In contrast, when we believe in His promises, our focus is no longer on the things of this world. We see the distant view—the eternity, the greatness of all divine reality. That is when we begin to comprehend who God really is.

The psalmist understood this reality when he wrote, "Whom have I in heaven but you? And earth has nothing I desire besides you" (Ps. 73:25, NIV). When our hearts are surrendered to God through the Holy Spirit, we no longer put our faith in our own abilities, but we trust in God. Isaiah 2:22 says, "Sever yourselves from such a man, whose breath is in his nostrils; for of what account is he?"

When we are centered on God, we have a fuller, deeper understanding of how much we need the Lord, and we are able to worship Him for His power and majesty. As we continually seek His heart, the things of this world are put in proper perspective, and we can enjoy them as we align ourselves with Him.

When we truly surrender to God in repentance and faith, we hand over our egos, our independence, our desires, and our worries about the future to Him. It is not easy to give up this control. As human beings we like to be in charge of our lives. And the world tells us that we should be in control. Yet when we cultivate relationship with God, He shows us our pride and helps us humble ourselves in His presence. Then we begin to see God as we ought. When we see life through God's eyes, we understand that His presence alone can satisfy our hearts. He will provide for us all that we need to fulfill His will for our lives. And as we learn more and more to trust implicitly in Him, we begin to find deep satisfaction and fulfillment in His love. That is when we are learning to fulfill the chief purpose of man, as the *Westminster Shorter Catechism* states: "to glorify God, and to enjoy Him for ever."

PEACE BEYOND COMPREHENSION

Let's look at a rubber band. It is either at ease in your hand or stretched by your fingers. And if it is stretched too tightly, it can break. In our psyches we may frequently feel like that stretched rubber band. We are at the breaking point because we are busy trying to do things by our own power. And when we are trying to be in control, basically we are caught up in the sin of selfishness. At that point we are stretched and tense like an overextended rubber band. We are not at peace, and we do not have the joy that comes from a relationship with God. We are acting like a three-year-old who wants to do it all by himself. And just as parents often do, God will let us fall to teach us that we need His divine presence and help continually working in our lives.

This brings us back to the Holy Spirit's work of felicity in our hearts—God's tranquility personified. The way to a peaceful life is to be surrendered and resting in the Lord. If we rest totally in Him, we are not stretched like a rubber band. If we give ourselves totally to Him to do His work, we are at ease. This comes by resting in His Word—in the promises He spoke by His mouth to our hearts. If we are busy praying and praising His majesty, we are at peace because we are where the Lord wants us to be, doing what He created us to do. We are filled with His tranquility.

Certainly we can think we have found happiness and joy while living in sin, but it is a false happiness and joy. With every ungodly activity we are stretched tighter and tighter when we sense our guilt as we seek our own pleasure. Instead, we need to seek God and be at rest in His love, which brings us genuine felicity.

Snow skiing, which I have enjoyed, can be a picture of our lives that are surrendered to God. In skiing, when you are ready to make a turn, you lower yourself and look downhill. Your knees go down into the hill, your feet go down an edge, and your entire body drops. This is called anticipation. You simply look down the hill with your whole body dropping and ready. Depending on the slope to carry you down the hill is like depending on the Lord. When you learn to yield to the slope, skiing becomes easy, and you expend much less effort. You can ski down the slope through the first turn with ease. When that turn is done, you get ready to anticipate the next one and prepare yourself for getting through it. When you learn to go from one state of anticipation to another, you glide through the turns, and the skiing is fun and easy.

How do we apply that to our daily lives? When we go through the "turns" of our lives with God, in a state of anticipation, believing in His promises, then it is easy to ski through the smooth terrain. And when we follow the pull of His gravity, we can negotiate the rough spots more easily as well. Yielding to Him to carry us fills us with joy that His presence is our help.

The psalmist describes this place of resting in the Lord beautifully in Psalm 131: "LORD, my heart is not haughty, nor my eyes lofty. Neither do I concern myself with great matters, nor with things too profound for me. Surely I have calmed and quieted my soul, like a weaned child with his mother; like a weaned child is my soul within me" (vv. 1–2).

When we are yielded to God, we have no agenda other than resting in the Lord and listening to Him. We seek the Holy Spirit, through faith and prayer, to dominate our direction. We do not try to manipulate what happens. We ask the Holy Spirit to determine our time, our mood, and our action. We just say, "Holy Spirit, my life is Yours. I'm going to anticipate Your presence in my life and be responsive to Your direction today."

Do not be anxious about anything, but in every situation, by prayer and petition, with thanksgiving, present your requests to God. And the peace of God, which transcends all understanding, will guard your hearts and your minds in Christ Jesus.

—PHILIPPIANS 4:6–7, NIV

There is a lot of talk about burnout in today's world, especially concerning the way it affects mothers, fathers, nurses, doctors, teachers, or caregivers. But when we trust in God's faithfulness, we feel less stress in the rigorous demands of life. By worshipping God's majesty and feeling His joy, we find God's enablement to face all life's challenges. We are not inactive or passive; we are active—even energetic—in our dependency on God. This dependency on Him, resting in His redemption, is the key to a joy-filled life.

One of the great spiritual lessons the famous missionary Hudson Taylor learned while on the mission field in China was where to rest his faith. While in England he learned to trust God for his needs without letting any other person know about them.[2] God honored this faith by providing for him all he needed for his life and ministry. He continued the principle of telling no one but God what he needed even while in China. However, when more and more young missionaries came to the field under his care and the needs were greater, he struggled with a need for greater faith. As he wrestled in his soul with this burden, God broke through to take him a step further in his relationship with God. God taught him to not trust in his own faith but to trust in God's *faithfulness*. It is in His faithfulness, not our faith, that we must put our trust. As Hudson learned to "feed on His faithfulness" (Ps. 37:3), his burden was lifted, and his joy returned. Resting in God's faithfulness is our source of peace and joy in the midst of all our trials. Let us listen to what the Spirit of God says: "He who calls you is faithful, who also will do it" (1 Thess. 5:24). "He who promised is faithful" (Heb. 10:23).

There are times when all of us feel that the burden of the cares of life is too heavy for us to bear. There are things about our lives that we cannot control. There is one answer to our dilemma, and that is to rest in and rejoice in God's faithfulness. The peace and joy that we find when we trust in Him are a sure pledge that His joy will continue to be perfected in us through all eternity. Let's pray.

> *Dear Lord, help me rest in You. Take my burdens, and let me enjoy the peace that comes with surrendering my life to You. Lord, let Your Holy Spirit fill every inch of me. Direct me! Convict me! Give me wisdom and strength! Let me know the sweet communion of my heart with Yours. Amen.*

OBEDIENCE

The apostle Paul, writing to the Philippians, describes Jesus as our role model, our perfect example of surrender to His Father.

> Have the same mindset as Christ Jesus: who, being in very nature God, did not consider equality with God something to be used to his own advantage; rather, he made himself nothing by taking the very nature of a servant, being made in human likeness. And being found in appearance as a man, he humbled himself by becoming obedient to death—even death on a cross!
> —Philippians 2:5–8, niv

So to live in obedience to the Father as Christ did, we must be humble, obedient, and ready to die to our own selfishness. That sounds like a difficult assignment. But this is not some dreary task that is placed upon us as Christians. The Holy Spirit works in our hearts to cause us to desire God above all other things. We are excited to love Him, believe in Him, obey Him, and serve Him. As we yield to the work of the Holy Spirit in our lives, we grow in our trust that comes from faith in His grace. Consider the rewards of this joyous mind-set. As we walk in obedience to God's Word, we have the assurance that God is in control of our lives. And we receive the benefits of enjoying a heart relationship with God, who loves us and will provide for us.

We must never think that we can learn to rest in God as a result of our own initiative, determination, or merit before God. Those attitudes reflect pride. We were all like sheep going astray when Jesus came and found us and laid us on His shoulders, rejoicing that He found His lost sheep. (See Luke 15:5.) We were following wrong voices and influences until He came and called us away from our self-destructive paths. Jesus said, "My sheep hear My voice, and I know them, and they follow Me" (John 10:27).

When we are resting in God, we are not full of pride or arrogance or selfishness. We have humbled ourselves to seek God and to obey His commands. Remember the fruit of the Spirit—love, joy, peace, patience, kindness, goodness, faithfulness, gentleness, and self-control? (See Galatians 5:22–23.) These are the divine spiritual qualities that fill us as we surrender ourselves to God and His will. These godly characteristics affect not only our relationship with God but also our relationships with others. Just like that married couple whose love spilled over into all areas of their lives, so the divine fruit of a life resting in God changes how we relate to others.

When we are resting in God, it is easier to give up the pretenses, pride, and self-righteousness that can destroy relationships with others. Instead, we respect others with godly dignity. We treat them with kindness and love. We can be transparent with them without a need to "cover things up."

The first couple, Adam and Eve, were free from shame and felt no need to hide anything from God or each other while they were living without sin. They were transparent with each other. They didn't hide their feelings. They enjoyed a truly intimate relationship. Only after they disobeyed the command of God did they hide themselves from Him and feel the need to cover themselves with clothes.

In the same way, we can be truly transparent in our relationships with others only when we are at rest in God and feel no need to hide behind false actions and attitudes.

CHAPTER 6

THE COMMITMENT TO
REMAIN AT REST

A LIFE OF INFINITE, glorious joy is a life that is continually resting in God. It is not always easy to remain at rest in God when facing difficult life situations or finding ourselves tempted by worldly desires, unhealthy emotions, and other depression and anxiety "triggers." That is why it is essential that we cultivate a lifestyle that involves spending time daily in quiet communion with our Lord, seeking Him in His Word and in prayer. The Holy Spirit aids our prayers and opens our understanding of the Scriptures, giving us power to face life's challenges in the peace and joy that comes from Christ alone. Jesus promised that the Holy Spirit would guide us into all truth (John 16:13) and that He would "glorify Me [Jesus], for He will take of what is Mine and declare it to you" (v. 14).

It is important to remember that just as life is a journey, lived one moment, hour, and day at a time, so is our posture of resting in God a progressive journey. Consider the analogy of the trapeze artist who must let go of one bar before he can start swinging on the next one. In that same way we must give up the "bars" of the world and our own will and desires so we can grab the "bars" of the Lord. We must learn more and more to desire the things of this world no longer but to find our true heart satisfaction in

Him alone. That will require our willingness to turn everything over to Him and trust Him with every area of our lives as well as life's challenges.

And just as a trapeze artist swings from bar to bar, so we must have the courage to let go of self-will and totally give ourselves to God. It is not a one-time event. It is a process that takes us through all kinds of situations in life as we build our relationship with God the Father, God the Son, and God the Holy Spirit. Consider the relationship you have built and are building with your spouse. That relationship did not happen overnight. There was the time you first met, the time you realized you were in love, and the time you truly committed yourself to that person. And even after that commitment, the two of you did not live in perfect unity all the time. You have had disagreements and misunderstandings as you have learned to love and understand each other. But when harmony and unity are restored, the love is greater; the joy at being back together and still being in love is sweeter. And you have gained a deeper understanding of your spouse.

That is a picture of our love relationship with God. The Scriptures say that "we love Him because He first loved us" (1 John 4:19). As we respond to His love, we commit our lives to Him. Yet we still struggle at times in our relationship with God. We find it difficult to give up our independence or personal desires that are not part of His plan for our holy living. Sometimes we may think there is be something better in the world than what He can provide. And too often these conflicts cause us to draw back from surrendering ourselves fully to God.

A LESSON IN TRUST

To remain in a resting posture with Christ, we will need to pass many lessons that will deepen our trust in Him. The Scriptures are filled with examples of those who have faced the difficulty of staying consistently surrendered to God's will for their lives.

One example in the Old Testament is the story of King Asa (2 Chron. 14–16.) When Asa began his reign, he was a great warrior and religious reformer. He trusted God for great things and had found God to be faithful in doing things beyond what Asa could ask or think. For example, he prayed for help for his nation against a powerful enemy: "LORD, there is no one like you to help the powerless against the mighty. Help us, LORD our God, for we rely on you, and in your name we have come against this vast army. LORD, you are our God; do not let mere mortals prevail against you" (2 Chron. 14:11, NIV). God answered his prayer, and Asa and his troops were victorious in battle.

But then Asa's kingdom was threatened by the king in the north of Israel, Baasha. Rather than trusting God, Asa cut a deal with the king of Syria to help them win this battle. He forgot that with God nothing shall be impossible. The prophet Hanani rebuked Asa for relying on Syria rather than on the Lord to conquer his enemy. The king was so angry he put the prophet in chains and continued to turn away from God. What did Hanani tell him?

> For the eyes of the LORD range throughout the earth to strengthen those whose hearts are fully committed to him.
>
> —2 CHRONICLES 16:9, NIV

The prophet called on Asa to remember God's love and power that He would show to those with hearts committed to Him. The king forgot how God provided for him in the previous battle and turned from his trust in God to put trust in man. He forgot that God delights to show Himself strong on behalf of those whose hearts are set on Him.

The message of the prophet was that God watched over and strengthened those "whose hearts are fully committed to him." Other translations read those "whose heart is perfect toward him" or "whose heart is loyal to Him." There is no substitute in our relationship with God for fully committing our lives into His loving hands. The Hebrew word translated "committed" is from the root verb, *shalom*, which means "peace, friendship—with God especially in covenant relationship." It is significant that it is also translated as "safety."[1] There can be no peace or safety without fully committing our hearts to God.

The word *shalom* is used again when Nehemiah rebuilt the walls of Jerusalem. He *shalomed* the walls, meaning he completed them. (See Nehemiah 6:15.) Those whose hearts are "shalomed" toward God are committed to, or loyal toward, Him. They are at peace—shalom—with God. When we trust not in our own strength but fix our sights on God's majesty and His great love for us, we have joyous, rested hearts that trust and depend on Him and believe in His promises.

> My God and my King, may my heart never forget Your promises, and may I be transformed through surrender to You.

LESSONS LEARNED FROM DAILY LIFE

Just as King Asa was drawn away from a relationship with God, so we face temptations in our lives to do the same. Often we find ourselves lured by the things and ways of this world. We get diverted in our walk with God, and we lose our joy in Him. Our focus shifts from God to ourselves, and we try to take back what we once surrendered to Him.

Why does this happen? Sometimes things are going well in our lives, and we begin to depend on these happy circumstances to satisfy our hearts. Then we forget to trust in Him and begin to think that we can actually take the credit for the good in our lives.

Or sometimes we get caught up in our daily troubles. We get so focused on them that they pull us down deeper and deeper, and we forget to seek God. A rested heart feels true joy in God's presence. But there are times when we feel God is far away. We face disappointments and wonder why God allowed it. There is a proverb that explains this dilemma: "Hope deferred makes the heart sick, but when the desire comes, it is a tree of life" (Prov. 13:12). All of us have had goals or hopes for our lives that have not materialized. But our hearts get sick when we get wrapped up in the disappointment and grief of that failed hope. Then, unless we take our grief to God and commit our way to Him, we will begin to walk down a path of bitterness, resentment, and self-pity because of that loss. We did not get what we wanted, and we sulk about it. That is fertile ground for depression to take root.

There is no room for God in that mind-set. We are not resting in redemption. We are selfish and want to wallow in our misery. Then the Spirit of God moves within us, and we realize the distance between our hearts and our God. We are lonely and frustrated. We see once again that we cannot rely on ourselves. If we turn to God and determine to trust His love for us, believing that He is our portion in this life and our all in all, we will once again know the joy of total commitment to Him. And the joy of that reunion with His presence fills us again. We experience what the psalmist did when he wrote:

> You turned my wailing into dancing; you removed my sackcloth and clothed me with joy.
>
> —PSALM 30:11, NIV

Dear Lord, help me every day to examine myself and surrender every area of my life to You. For in Your loving arms I am filled, not with the delights of this world but with Your joy.

DOING OR BEING?

Is there someone you know who is one of the first people to get up, get organized, and start moving vigorously, churning from one task to another? He finds great satisfaction in simply *doing* tasks at hand. Maybe that person is you. If you're not careful, all the energy that goes to completing tasks distracts you from relying on the Lord to fill you with His presence.

Whether we are the first ones out of bed in the morning or not, we must all remember that everything we do in our tasks and errands and duties is focused on temporal activities. Starting our day by spending time with the Lord in communion with

His heart of love will focus our minds on the *eternal* realities of walking with Him and resting in His love. The eternal things are unseen. As we focus on them by faith, we have the pleasures of God in our hearts to help us rest in His love. In that place of divine rest, we will find that we enjoy the love of God in our works as well.

The Gospel of Luke tells a story about two sisters with a similar conflict between actions of the hands and attitudes of the heart. Jesus and His disciples stopped at the home of Mary and Martha to visit and eat. Martha scurried around getting things ready for the meal, and she became agitated because Mary just sat at Jesus' feet, listening to what He said. Martha asked Him, "Lord, don't you care that my sister has left me to do the work by myself? Tell her to help me!" (Luke 10:40, NIV). Then Jesus answered her:

> "Martha, Martha," the Lord answered, "you are worried and upset about many things, but few things are needed—or indeed only one. Mary has chosen what is better, and it will not be taken away from her."
> —LUKE 10:41–42, NIV

There are a lot of people like Martha. They are geared toward getting tasks accomplished, checking them off to-do lists, and moving on to some other task. Those people who love God and relate to the "Martha" approach to life are not hopeless. They can live a committed life resting in His redemption as long as they remember what is most important: they must surrender themselves daily to seek God and let Him prioritize their to-do lists.

For example, a Martha might set a goal of reading through the whole Bible. If she remembers to look into the Lord's eyes as she reads, she can become a Mary. She has to ask herself whether she really looks for Christ in her reading or if she is too busy getting the job done—just reading the Bible through. Is she asking the Lord to fill her with His presence as she reads the Scriptures, or is she too intent on her goal of completing the task?

We are either asking Him to reveal His life within us, or we have diverted our gaze from Him. We need to stop and listen to God, to work out a closeness with Him that helps us surrender ourselves daily to Him. Let's pray.

> *Lord, teach me as a Martha to become more like Mary. Teach me to not try to prove myself by tasks and deeds, however good they might be. Teach me to come close to You in meekness. Teach me to be open and honest, and show me that nothing matters other than You.*

SEEKING WHAT WE WANT OR WHAT GOD WANTS?

> A heart at peace gives life to the body, but envy rots the bones.
>
> —PROVERBS 14:30, NIV

Coveting may be one of the biggest things that keeps us from the kind of rest in God that brings peace to our souls and spirits. The dictionary defines *covet* as "to wish for greatly or with envy."[2] For Christians, it means that our hearts desire something more than we desire relationship with Jesus.

The Scriptures declare an amazing insight into the reason the Pharisees wanted a pagan ruler, Pilate, to crucify Christ. They declare Pilate knew "that for envy they had delivered him" (Matt. 27:18, KJV). They were upset that all the people were going after Jesus. They coveted the power and the love of the people that Jesus received because He was totally committed to do the will of His Father. So in envy the Pharisees delivered Christ to be crucified. We must not allow covetousness or envy to separate us from our godly relationship of resting in the Lord. If we do, we will not have true peace and joy.

In all facets of life, we can destroy ourselves by wanting the wrong things or even too much of what we already have. We want when we need not. Our wants keep us from having the joy of relationships that are godly—a godly relationship with each other and a godly relationship with our Redeemer.

People who covet a lot of things are frequently anxious about everything and oversensitive to everything that happens to them—in their personal lives, their work, and their relationships. Some people even destroy their marriages by wanting other things more than a healthy, loving relationship with their spouses, especially if they become involved in other relationships. Caring too much about the things of this world will definitely have a negative impact on our heart relationship with God as well as other facets of our lives. Mark 4:19 says, "The worries of this life, the deceitfulness of wealth and the desires for other things come in and choke the word, making it unfruitful" (NIV).

Perhaps you see this inner, destructive motive of coveting in your own envious attitudes, in your relationships with colleagues, in interpersonal relationships. It destroys your productivity, your peace within your workplace, and everything else in your life because you are envious of someone else. Instead of being thankful for what you have and feeling grateful and blessed, you feel envious to the point of negating your own place in life and, certainly, your communion with Christ. Envy of worldly things takes away from your surrender to Him because it prevents you from resting in the Lord. It keeps you in the world rather than focused on the eternal. It keeps you from expressing faith and joy.

The things you covet also keep you from enjoying the things you have. There is an old story about four cows in a field. The field was fenced off into four sections, and each cow had its own section to enjoy. Yet each cow had its neck through the fence, trying to get the grass in another cow's section. That is a graphic picture of the foolishness of covetousness. Coveting causes us anxiety and robs us of the pleasure of things we have been given to enjoy.

The rested life doesn't focus on *things*. When we believe God's promises, we are filled with joy, peace, and righteousness. An abandoned faith puts God first, and then we are able to more fully enjoy the things He has given us, expressing our gratitude for all we have received from His hand.

The story Jesus tells about a rich man and a poor beggar, Lazarus, who eats crumbs from the rich man's table, is a perfect example of the folly of making *things* our goal for life. In this story Jesus tells us that there is no correlation between what we have on earth and what we have when we die. Even though Lazarus had nothing and was physically suffering on earth, he had a relationship with God. And while the rich man had everything, he was proud and arrogant with no thought of God. But their positions were reversed when they died. Lazarus was carried to the peaceful rest to dwell at the right side of Abraham; the rich man lifted up his face in torment in hell (Luke 16:19–26).

Does this mean that if we have worldly goods, we will spend eternity in hell? Not at all. Our possessions do not matter to God; it is our attitude toward them that matters. What we need is to live a life that is not set on gaining worldly goods but is pursuing relationship with God in abandoned faith and a surrendered spirit. Lazarus had nothing to prevent him from resting in the Lord; the rich man did. Sometimes we let our possessions or desires keep us from turning to God. Then, when we do turn to God, we struggle with surrendering those things to Him.

We must remember to keep our attitude toward earthly possessions in check, guarding our lives against the sin of covetousness. If we begin to believe our possessions make us important, we put our trust in them and become proud and arrogant in thinking our own abilities are enough to provide our needs. But if we remember that everything we have comes from God, we can keep our focus on Him and live a life that is surrendered to His will.

> *Dear God, may my eyes never lose sight of You, that I can focus on eternal treasures and not the possessions of this world. Show me my pride daily so it does not hinder me from walking with You!*

THE ANXIETY "DISEASE"

Anxiety is one of the greatest hindrances to resting in God's redemption. We must embrace God's Rx for the destructive emotion of anxiety that affects every life situation we encounter. In the medical profession doctors see patients who frequently worry themselves sick. This type of worry escalates into anxiety and becomes one of the worst diseases to treat. It destroys people by destroying the quality of their lives, the length of their lives—every part of their lives.

There is only one answer for a life filled with anxiety—surrendering ourselves to God in absolute faith in His grace. Such a faith declares that He is our answer to everything. Resting in the power of the resurrection that redeems us is the answer to all. How often we need to pray this prayer:

> Dear Lord, keep me strong in my faith in You and Your grace. Help me put my faith in You when I am more inclined to trust in myself. Help me to not be distracted by the trials of daily life but instead to rely on Your love and strength. Keep me focused on the big picture of who You are and what You are going to do for me!

A CRITICAL SPIRIT

A heart filled with love is essential for us to truly rest in God. But sometimes our pride gets the better of us, and we forfeit our peace and joy in His redemption by becoming critical of others. We can develop a habit of criticizing others to build up ourselves. When that happens, we have lost sight of God's love for us and the great value He places on our lives. There is no higher affirmation than to know the peace of God and enjoy His presence as we walk in His will for our lives.

When we try to measure ourselves by others' success or standing in society, and so on, we have lost sight of our true personhood as a child of God. We are not walking in the commandments of God to love Him with all our hearts and to love others as ourselves (Matt. 22:37–40). Instead of loving others as He has loved us, we become their accusers rather than intercessors seeking God for their good. When we begin to criticize others, we end up destroying ourselves along with the many things that are most important to us, particularly those who are closest to us.

> *Lord, help me to follow Your example of love and humility. Keep me from being critical for the sake of my own ego, and help me to act with kindness, not pride.*

DISCUSSION ❧ QUESTIONS

Describe an area of your life that has been a struggle in your relationship with God, something you have found yourself needing to surrender to Him over and over again.

....

....

....

What happens when you take that area back again? Do you notice a difference mentally, emotionally, or physically?

....

....

....

How does slowing down to view things from an eternal perspective change what you want out of relationships, situations, or your life in general?

....

....

....

Ask the Holy Spirit to shine a light on areas of your heart where you have allowed negative emotions, such as worry, anxiety, and a critical spirit, to take over. Write a prayer asking for His help to replace these harmful emotions with His love.

....

....

CHAPTER 7

RESTING OR
RELIGIOUS?

URRENDER. SUBMISSION. SELFLESSNESS. These are godly traits that characterize our love relationship with God. When we submit ourselves to God, we find ourselves filled with joy. When we surrender our egos and independence to God, we find ourselves filled with glorious, abundant joy. We are at peace with ourselves because we have found peace in God. Then we are full of joy because we love God and depend on Him—not on ourselves.

However, let us never forget that it is not our works or religious activities but receiving and resting in the love of God that is the fountain of our inner life toward God. Jesus said,

> Whoever drinks of the water that I shall give him will never thirst. But the water that I shall give him will become in him a fountain of water springing up into everlasting life.
>
> —JOHN 4:14

Earlier we talked about how the temptations and problems of the world can lure us away from a rested life. But some of our fiercest struggles are sometimes a result of being followers of

Christ—when we get so busy *doing* all the right things that we forget to be still and listen to Christ in communion with Him through prayer and His Word. That temptation to busyness with *good* works robs us of Christ's peace and joy because our attention and energies are focused on religious activities.

Within all of us there is a tug between the rested spirit and a religious one. Now, on the surface having a religious spirit sounds like a good thing. But having a religious spirit means we are following the religious culture, going through the motions of having faith in God but not really committing our lives to seeking Him and cultivating a heart relationship with Him. When we function only in a religious spirit, we do not truly love Him or believe in His promises. We appear externally as if we were religious, doing good deeds or belonging to certain organizations. A rested heart that is following after Jesus allows God to change us from presenting an external appearance of religiosity to living in fellowship with Christ that is reflected in a life of joy and love that emanates from our hearts and is visible in our actions.

The Old Testament gives us many examples that illustrate the problems with a religious spirit. Chapter 4 of 1 Samuel tells us about a series of battles between the Israelites and the Philistines. In one battle the Israelites lost four thousand men. So they sent the message back to the city of Shiloh: bring the ark of the covenant to the battlefield. The Israelites planned to carry it into the next battle, hoping God would bless them because the ark was present. That was their religious tradition.

The ark contained the tables of the law. But it also had an atonement cover (or mercy seat) to proclaim that there is forgiveness with God. The presence of that cover made it a type of God's throne representing grace. So the ark was not just a physical presence or religious symbol; it was a symbol of God's covenant with His people and their commitment to Him.

There was a holy precedent for carrying this holy symbol of God into battle. For example, God told Joshua at the battle of Jericho to have priests march at the front of his army carrying the ark. When they obeyed God's command, the walls of Jericho collapsed, and Joshua's army was victorious (Josh. 6:1–21).

But when the Israelites decided to use the ark in their battle against the Philistines, they were not following God's command; they were just looking for an edge in the fight in enlisting a religious tradition. They wanted the outward blessing of battle—victory—without an inward devotion to God. Bringing the ark to the battle was an outward and showy attempt to manipulate God. This was the religious spirit at its worst—a spirit that relies on false actions, not heartfelt faith. Not only was what they did wrong; it was done with wrong motives.

The Israelites must have been surprised at the outcome. Not only did they lose the battle, but also thirty thousand men were killed, and the ark was captured by the Philistines. The whole experience was summarized in the word *ichabod*, which means "the glory is departed" or the Lord has departed from Shiloh and all of Israel with the capture of the ark.[1]

We need to examine our own lives. Have we set God before us to love and obey, or are we using religious tradition to help us achieve our own goals? The godly way to consider it is set down by the psalmist.

> I keep my eyes always on the LORD. With him at my right hand, I will not be shaken.
>
> —PSALM 16:8, NIV

Dear God, let me not be shaken but have my eyes fixed firmly on You. Let my actions speak for my beliefs, and let me not have false attitudes and activities that do not reflect Your joy.

A SELFISH SPIRIT

When we have a religious spirit, we are focused more on ourselves and what God can do for us than we are on His majesty and grace. We are not cultivating relationship with Him that seeks to know His will and what we are called to do for Him. We start presenting Him with lists of demands; we do not want to give our lives to Him as faithful servants. In short, we are selfish and self-centered. We want to do only what is convenient for us to reach our goals. Jesus warned about this attitude when He lectured the Pharisees, quoting from the words of the prophet Isaiah.

> These people honor me with their lips, but their hearts are far from me. They worship me in vain; their teachings are merely human rules.
> —MATTHEW 15:8–9, NIV

When we are governed by a religious spirit, our human desire to be independent takes over. We start thinking that we know best. We start relying on our own decisions and abilities rather than on the limitless power of the almighty God.

Our hearts are not in the right place. We may go through the motions of believing or follow all the religious rules, but that does not get us anywhere. Rather than being focused on ourselves, we need to follow the advice of the psalmist.

> Look to the LORD and his strength; seek his face always.
> —PSALM 105:4, NIV

Father, I mean to trust in You and let You have control of my life. But often I fail. May my joy in You keep me strong.

THE FOLLY OF PRIDE

Humility isn't something that comes naturally to people. We want to be proud of who we are, what we accomplish, and what we own. God does not dwell with those who have proud hearts.

> Though the LORD be high, yet hath he respect unto the lowly: but the proud he knoweth afar off.
> —PSALM 138:6, KJV

A rested heart requires purity and separation from our base human attitudes, which are lurking within us regardless of how close we are to the Lord. We are frequently tempted to think we have the answer to a situation. In fact, in our own egotism, sometimes we think we are "the answer" and frequently do not turn to Christ to seek His will in the matter.

True humility results from submitting our lives to God and worshipping Him. We are not humble by nature. Humility is not something we can decide to acquire. We become humble only as we pursue our Lord and love and follow Him. And our submission to Him becomes all-consuming—affecting every part of our body, permeating us, and directing us. Humility is reflected in our lives when we are molded by the Holy Spirit.

Dear God, keep my arrogance in check, and remind me who You are, how much You love me, and how You will continually provide for me.

THE TYRANNY OF LEGALISM

One of the strong tenants of a religious spirit is legalism. A legalistic spirit causes us to lose our focus on God and focus rather on following man-made rules and regulations. To our natural thinking, following rules is easier than trying to seek God and follow His will. When we walk in the path of legalism, we quit trusting in Him, and we start trying to control our own lives. The tyranny of our self-effort to be righteous always leads to failure in life.

Only the Holy Spirit can work in us to break this religious mind-set. When we focus on rules and regulations, we no longer follow God's greatest commandment: "Love the LORD your God with all your heart, with all your soul, and with all your strength" (Deut. 6:5). Instead of love, we follow "law" and are filled with a spirit of legalism. The apostle Paul warned us in 2 Corinthians of how lethal this love of rules and regulations can be.

> He has made us competent as ministers of a new cov-
> enant—not of the letter [or law] but of the Spirit; for the
> letter kills, but the Spirit gives life.
> —2 CORINTHIANS 3:6, NIV

Jesus battled those with a spirit of legalism during His ministry here on earth. He criticized them for following minor external rules and tradition rather than focusing on loving God with their hearts. This religious spirit with its dominating rules kept the Jewish leaders from being surrendered to God. They failed to adore and praise God. Jesus preached the necessity of a rested heart that truly surrenders to the love of God.

Jesus, remind me that You must be my focus. Let me dwell in You and be Your child for eternity.

REBELLION VS. REDEMPTION

C. S. Lewis would often ask intellectuals to imagine, if they could, a God who would provide for them, love them, and be their constant source of strength. Then he would philosophize with them on whether that was a good thing or a bad thing.

It is a good thing to think we were created by a divine Person, Elohim the Creator, and to consider that He had a design for us because He loves us. Yet our personal independence and rebellion keep us from accepting that divine reality. To accept the fact of a loving Creator requires that we determine what we want our relationship to be to Him.

When we are self-centered, we do not want any other "being," no matter how noble or legitimate his claims, to interfere with our lives. We refuse to look at life from eternity's perspective; in that sense, we live all our lives in rebellion against God.

There is another way of looking at it. Each of us develops, to a greater or lesser extent, a passive-aggressive personality as we grow up. For example, when your parents told you to sit down, you sat down passively, but you were still "standing up" on the inside. That is a picture of rebellion. When we begin to follow God and receive redemption through Christ, we receive His forgiveness of our rebellion and begin to exchange it for love of God and others. Then we learn to serve one another and submit to one another in love.

Without yielding to the work of the Holy Spirit in our hearts through redemption, that rebellion in us can evolve into defiance that insists on pursuing its selfish agenda. We insist on always having our own way, which makes us difficult to live with. This selfish rebellion can become manipulative, become destructive, and leave us feeling frustrated, unhappy, and angry.

We develop in our relationship with God as we struggle to give up our pride and independence and rest in Him. As we learn to live in His presence, He empowers us to be freed from our mental, physical, and sinful rebellion. As redeemed children of God, we become one with Him.

We must continually seek God in order to grow in our relationship with God. Central to all our growth in God is the realization that Jesus must be our chief portion in this life—our greatest joy—and that the joy of the Lord is our strength. The following prayer is not one we can pray just once or twice; we need to pray daily.

> *Heavenly Father, even though I am Your child, I do not want to be childish. Help me grow and mature in my love, and help me surrender continually to You.*

DISCUSSION 🌿 QUESTIONS

Think of times when your selfishness, pride, and rebellion have caused severed relationships with God or with others. Describe what you've learned from those situations.

....

....

Do you believe that God truly loves you, provides for you, and is your complete source of strength? Or do you strive to make your way through life as a result of your own efforts?

....

....

What is your reason for living? (As you grow and mature in your Christian life, the Lord should become the greatest portion of your life.)

....

....

How does the Holy Spirit help you grow in your relationship with the Lord?

....

....

CHAPTER 8

RESTORED
TO JOY

A s I HAVE mentioned, life in Christ requires a daily discipline to allow us to remain resting in God. Sometimes we fail. Our desire for independence and control takes over, we forget God's promises, and we turn away from Him. When that happens, our lives can become consumed with bitterness, hatred, frustration, and anger. We need to understand that we are living in sin when we are not living in God's presence, seeking to do His will for our lives.

But when we do fail, God gives us a path back to Him, a way to restore the precious inner relationship we once enjoyed with our Savior. It involves simply confessing our sin and repenting. When we humble ourselves in His presence, we experience overwhelming joy in renewing our communion with Him. The psalmist understood this pathway back to God.

> Create in me a pure heart, O God, and renew a steadfast spirit within me. Do not cast me from your presence or take your Holy Spirit from me. Restore to me the joy of your salvation and grant me a willing spirit, to sustain me.
>
> —PSALM 51:10–12, NIV

In this psalm David writes of the joy of coming back into a right relationship with God. When we confess our sins and repent, we experience overwhelming joy in feeling His presence again. We are filled with wonder and awe at His grace, and we worship His greatness and majesty. Separation from God means sadness. Reunion with Him means joy and gladness.

Confessing our sins is an important step on the path of a rested heart. When we confess, we admit that we have sinned against God's love. Jesus tells a story in Luke 15 to illustrate this. A son asked his father for his inheritance, took the money, and traveled far from home. He squandered all the money, and then he was forced to look for work.

He could find only one job—feeding pigs. He realized his working conditions were worse than those of his father's workers. He decided to go home and ask his father to treat him as he would any other hired hand. "The son said to him, 'Father, I have sinned against heaven and against you. I am no longer worthy to be called your son'" (Luke 15:21, NIV).

But the father was not angry that his son had wasted his money and time. He did not take him back as an employee and say, "I told you so," or lecture him. Instead, he rejoiced that his son had come home. He said, "Bring the fattened calf and kill it. Let's have a feast and celebrate. For this son of mine was dead and is alive again; he was lost and is found" (Luke 15:23–24, NIV).

Too often we are like that son. We rely on our own abilities and skills, and we do not trust in the Lord with all our hearts. We are ungrateful when we receive blessings from God, and we do not give Him the credit. And we do not admit that we are living in this sinful attitude. Our actions speak louder than our false words. They show that we do not believe God is worthy of our loyalty. We have turned from a rested spirit to a false pride and trust in our own strength and understanding.

As the prodigal son confessed his unworthiness, so we must admit that we have dishonored God. We do not confess because we were caught at our sin or were embarrassed by it. We must confess because we have offended the God who loves us. As Proverbs 28:13 says, "He who covers his sins will not prosper, but whoever confesses and forsakes them will have mercy." We must be honest, we must be specific, and we must be thorough when we confess our sins to God.

> *Father, I am such a rebellious child. Lord, my motives were from love of myself, not love and praise of You.*

SEEKING GOD'S FORGIVENESS

After we have confessed our sins, we must ask God's forgiveness: "Oh, pity and forgive me by the blood of Christ." When we ask His forgiveness, we surrender ourselves to Him and are cleansed. Then nothing stands between our Redeemer and us.

Then we must rise up and praise Him for forgiveness. We believe it. We embrace it. We delight in it. "I'm forgiven! I'm clean before the Lord!" After all, God has promised He would forgive us. It is His desire for us to ask. First John 1:9 says, "If we confess our sins, He is faithful and just to forgive us our sins and to cleanse us from all unrighteousness." We treat God as a liar if we do not truly believe we are forgiven and rejoice in His redemption. Then we have the joy of being free from the guilt of sin. Until we seek His forgiveness, we cannot have that kind of joy. That forgiveness, that freedom is essential to our well-being, body, soul, and spirit.

Because we are human, we all seem to wander right back into things that we should not do; we deviate from His standard. So asking forgiveness is not just a one-time event. We need to constantly be aware of our thoughts, our actions, our lack of action, and anything else in which we fail. Paul describes this state of sinful living in Romans 14:23: "Whatever is not from faith is sin." Let us not be of anything other than faith in Him. We should have no agenda other than seeking to please Him, to fellowship with Him, to serve Him, and to seek forgiveness when we sin.

Dear Lord, forgive me when I stray from You and lose sight of Your glory, majesty, and love. I praise You for Your mercy, grace, and forgiveness, which free me from the bondage of sin.

THE JOY OF REPENTANCE

If you repent, I will restore you.

—JEREMIAH 15:19, NIV

Repentance is bittersweet. The sweetness comes from God's forgiveness, welcome, and acceptance of us because of Jesus' death on the cross. This is the eternal comfort that only God can give. This is the joy of knowing God as my heavenly Father. The bitterness is the memory, shame, guilt, and sorrow for having offended God. The bitterness of sin is God's means of bringing us to seek Him. We become so miserable that we cannot stand to be alienated from God any longer. Once we come to God through the Lord Jesus, the sweetness overshadows the bitterness and gives way to joy unspeakable and full of glory. (See 1 Peter 1:8.)

When we confess our sins and seek God's forgiveness, we realize who we are and how majestic God is. We see the awesome power of His grace, that He would continue to love us and restore and uphold a relationship with us even though we sin against Him. There is a sweet brokenness that accompanies the tears of remorse—the melting and relenting of the soul returning to God, lamenting its former unkindness. "A broken and a contrite heart—these, O God, You will not despise" (Ps. 51:17). This means that God does not despise our brokenness. On the contrary, He delights to embrace a broken heart with His love. And He restores to us the joy of our salvation.

But Jesus does not just forgive us. He is as determined to make us holy as He is to forgive us. Titus 2:14 says that Christ "gave Himself for us, that He might redeem us from every lawless deed and purify for Himself His own special people, zealous for good works." This was His intention on the cross. He was not only saying, "Father, redeem them, forgive them, and pardon them." He was saying as well, "Father, make them holy, purify them, and bring them to a special relationship of loyalty and faithfulness." These characteristics describe a special people who desire more than all else to live near to God and to live according to His Word. May God make us such a people!

Father, take my sins, burdens, and my selfishness, and forgive me. Help me to live a life of purity before Your eyes. Enable me to worship You and enjoy Your peace and joy.

DISCUSSION QUESTIONS

Pause right now to examine your heart for things you need to ask God to forgive. Write a prayer asking for His forgiveness.

....

....

....

How does unforgiven sin affect your relationship with God?

....

....

....

Describe the difference between the conviction of the Holy Spirit and condemnation, which comes only from the enemy.

....

....

....

What does becoming holy mean to you?

....

....

....

CHAPTER 9

WORSHIP
AND JOY

*Blessed are the people who know the joyful
sound! They walk, O LORD, in the light of Your countenance. In Your name they rejoice all day long,
and in Your righteousness they are exalted.*

—PSALM 89:15–16

HAVE YOU EVER almost worshipped someone, such as a teacher when you were in second grade, the homecoming king or queen, or maybe even a movie star or singer? Though "creature worship" is foolish and wrong, it is often an overwhelming, uncontrollable devotion, even a passion. We would give up everything for that person, and we would do everything in our power to be just like him or her.

Now compare that with worshipping God. It is a much greater relationship than anything we experience with another human being because when we believe in God, we begin to see His power and glory and grace. We behold His countenance, and we are overwhelmed by His majesty. Worship is a summary of our entire response to God, who is the beginning and the end, the Maker of heaven and earth, our Creator and Redeemer.

All things are of God, all things are through God, and all things are sustained by the breadth of His might. His knowledge is without bounds. His wisdom is infinite. His riches are immense and inexhaustible. His majesty is awe-inspiring.

"In Him we live and move and have our being" (Acts 17:28). We open our eyes and know He is there. He has rained down blessings from heaven upon the earth where He has placed us. This rich and well-furnished world provides all our necessities. God's love and power are infinitely greater than any need that we may have of Him. He is above our reach. He is above our conceptions; we cannot comprehend Him. Yet when we surrender our lives to God and believe in His promises, we find our ultimate existence and purpose in Him.

Once we are in God's presence, we cannot help but worship His majesty and praise Him. We also cannot help but find joy in God's grace and power. There is no other way to feel when we fall at the feet of the Master. We are in awe of the salvation and fellowship He bestows on all who trust in Him.

Indeed, the excellency of His nature creates the fires of worship, the desire to praise and glorify Him. Worship is not a pathway to something greater; it is an end in itself. The goal of worship is not to see what we can get out of it; the goal of worship is to exalt God. Worship is gladly reflecting to God the radiance of His worth. It is a spontaneous emotion that genuinely comes from the heart that has tasted His wonderful redemption and is resting in His love.

Father, You are Lord, and You are God. Let me fall at Your feet and worship You as my Maker, Redeemer, and Savior.

LOVE AND WORSHIP

Whatever we love, we praise. Whatever we love, we delight in and enjoy. But this love, this enjoyment, this delight, is incomplete until we can express it. We express our love and delight to

God by worshipping Him. He wants us to adore and worship and exalt Him. When we do that, we cannot help but be filled with joy. "I will praise You, O LORD, with my whole heart; I will tell of all Your marvelous works," Psalm 9:1 says.

John Piper, in his book *Desiring God*, calls this joy and pleasure in God "Christian hedonism."[1] We are satisfied with the excellency of God. We are overwhelmed with the joy of His fellowship. This is the feast of "Christian hedonism"—to be filled with eternal, spiritual, godly pleasures.

This "hedonistic" approach is the only humble approach because it comes with empty hands, depending totally upon God for our pleasures and acknowledging that He alone can satisfy the heart's longing to be happy. We love God and are filled with joy at being in His presence.

Jonathan Edwards said religious affections and charity, or love, are the fountain of true religion in the heart.[2] Anything other than that is false. Without this genuine affection and inclination of the soul, religion is dead. We worship God because we love Him and believe His promises.

Try starting each of your prayers by saying, "Lord, You loved me first, and I love You." This expresses the reality that your religion is based in affection. Edwards said, "True religion, in great part, consists in holy affections....The affections are no other than the...sensible exercises of the inclination and will of the soul."[3]

> Then I will go to the altar of God, to God, my joy and my delight. I will praise you with the lyre, O God, my God.
>
> —PSALM 43:4, NIV

If we love someone, we treat that person with appreciation, attention, tenderness, and honor. Husbands and wives must love and appreciate each other and care for each other; otherwise, they can get critical, selfish, negative, and judgmental. We must be appreciative in any relationship: with a friend, a coworker, a business partner, or a neighbor. It is essential for us to appreciate one another; otherwise, we cannot encourage, praise, intercede for, or love others.

Just as we are aware of the love in our relationships with those who really care for us, God is aware of how much we love and appreciate Him. Our worship of Him parallels how thankful we are for His grace, majesty, glory, sovereignty, and perfect will. From that love and thanksgiving comes a constant state of joy, worship, and prayer that permeates us. First Thessalonians 5:16–18 describes this constant state of being.

> Rejoice always, pray without ceasing, in everything give
> thanks; for this is the will of God in Christ Jesus for you.

When we are truly able to let all earthly concerns go, we can find ourselves in a "thanksgiving frenzy"—a time in our relationship with God when we are so filled with joy in His presence that we thank Him for everything we can think of; we are in a state of total abandonment to our faith in Him. We can sense how close we are to Him and how far away we have turned from our own personal needs. We are no longer wrapped up in ourselves; we are lifted up into His presence.

This is when we feel closer to God than we do at other times. We just thank Him, knowing our lack and His greatness. He is from the beginning of time and all through eternity, and yet He is at the center of our little lives. These thanksgiving frenzies can allow us to worship Him in a special way—we do not have to carry a tune or be a great theologian. We simply appreciate the Lord God Almighty.

Now, we cannot experience these thanksgiving frenzies all the time. But we should seek to be constantly in a state of faith, joy, and worship. We must remember to be focused on the Lord and thankful to Him for whatever happens. We can use various ways to stay focused—simply by saying Bible verses or praying. It is a matter of maintaining a constant flow of attention to God.

All of us should seek this attitude of faith, joy, and worship.

We must make it part of all our lives and realize it is the only important thing that we are doing at any time. Whether we are practicing our chosen profession, participating in the activities of our daily lives, or simply kneeling in prayer with no one watching, we need to be focused on God. God has so designed worship that we receive an immense satisfaction from exalting Him. This background of love and worship that meditates on His goodness and His love is essential to a peaceful, abundant, godly, and joyous life! May our hearts accelerate with joy as we pray.

Lord, I stand in awe of Your majesty, Your grace, and Your love. May I always honor You with all my thoughts, desires, and actions and always believe Your promises.

EXALTING GOD AND BEING EXALTED BY HIM

More than anything the Lord wants from us, He wants us to praise and worship Him and only Him, unconditionally and without reservations. He tells us this in the Old Testament. Speaking to Moses in Exodus 34:14, God said, "You shall worship no other god, for the LORD, whose name is Jealous, is a jealous God."

God said He would tolerate no rivals for the loyalty of the people of Israel. His name, or character, is Jealous. He demands that same kind of exclusive devotion from us. God wants what is rightfully His. How should we respond to Him, as our Creator and Redeemer? Praise should be given to God for who He is, so we lift Him up, or exalt Him.

It may seem strange that a God who is supposed to be all loving wants to be all exalted. But it is not a vain desire; He wants our worship because He gives Himself back to us when we worship Him. He asks us to exalt Him with everything we have, and with that exaltation we are lifted up. It is like a husband saying to his wife, "Sweetheart, you stick with me because I am determined to take care of you and bless you!"

God wants us to share in the demonstration of His glory, to

enjoy His glory, to give Him glory. Now, it might seem selfish to us that God wants our total devotion, worship, and faith. Yet that is exactly the way it is. It is simply the affirmation of the Creator for the created and the created for the Creator.

> Yours, O LORD, is the greatness, the power and the glory, the victory and the majesty; for all that is in heaven and in earth is Yours; Yours is the kingdom, O LORD, and You are exalted as head over all.
> —1 CHRONICLES 29:11

Jesus told us the greatest commandments are to "love the LORD your God with all your heart, with all your soul, and with all your mind" and "love your neighbor as yourself" (Matt. 22:37, 39). And while in worldly realms it may appear selfish, in godly terms it is the epitome of unselfishness. Maybe we should call it godly self-ishness. In godly selfishness we realize the best thing we can do is worship God and give worth to others. This godly selfishness benefits us, and it benefits others. What we gain is a closer rela-tionship with God, which helps everyone.

Human, or carnal, selfishness is something we maintain solely for ourselves. Godly selfishness is the only way to ascribe worth to God and to others. So worship is a self-advantageous thing: not only does it lift us up, but it also lifts up all the relationships around us.

Our highest good and joy come from keeping our focus on God in true worship. True worship is personal, real, and deeply satisfying. Our self enters into the greatest experience of our existence when we worship God.

In any relationship in which two people care about each other, each strives to make the other happier. That is true as we worship God out of our love for Him. We want to please Him and exalt Him. And as He is exalted, He cares to make us happy by giving us a closer relationship with Himself.

It is empty striving to think we can obtain the Spirit's joy and peace in any other way besides our exaltation of God. With our exaltation we accept a pearl of His presence, which is the greatest gift we can receive. That pearl of His presence gives us the fruit of the Spirit—love, joy, peace, patience, kindness, goodness, faithfulness, gentleness, and self-control—that comes from simply praising Him.

> *Lord God, as I worship You, change me. Fill me with true humility and love that I may better love You and serve those around me. Work this into my life by the power of Your Holy Spirit.*

DUTY OR LOVE?

You have crowned him with glory and honor.

—HEBREWS 2:7

Throughout the Bible we are told that we should crown the Lord with glory and honor. God desires honor and splendor to be given to Him freely in gratitude from our hearts for His love for us. The joy we experience in worshipping God cannot be experienced in any other act. C. S. Lewis said, "The very nature of Joy makes nonsense of our common distinction between having and wanting."[4] In other words, joy turns our having to into wanting to.

Love, not duty, strengthens us in our service and in our work for God. Let me explain with an example. If I come home on my wedding anniversary with a dozen red roses for my wife and she says, "My, you have these beautiful roses for me. Why did you do it?" Suppose I reply, "I did it because it is my duty. A man should have character and should give his wife roses for their anniversary." Such a response would not go over well. It would not make her heart glad. Nor does it make the Lord glad if we do everything merely out of duty.

Suppose a husband tells his wife, "Honey, I just want to be with you; I just want to hold your hands and be close to you. These red roses are just a token of how my heart feels—wanting to be as close as possible to you. Let's spend the day together." Most wives would respond very differently to an expression of love such as this one than they would to one of duty. It is not a husband's duty that pleases his wife but his joy and honor to be with her. Similarly, the Lord also wants our love rather than just our sense of duty. We need to delight in Him, and He will give us the request of our hearts—namely, the satisfaction and joy of the Holy Spirit.

Chuck Colson was a fabulous Christian and one of the greatest citizens of America. He expounded the gospel of Jesus Christ in a very courageous way. And he was faithful, fervent, and focused in His love for Christ, reflected through his work among our nation's prisons and in many other ways.

Several years ago Chuck was one of the speakers at a meeting and gave his usual talk about the duty of Christianity. He was a good lawyer, and he analyzed everything very well, discussing duty to God and country, duty to society, duty to our families, and many other duties that we as Christians need to recognize. He used many Scripture references, such as this one: "It is God himself who has made us what we are and given us new lives from Christ Jesus; and long ages ago he planned that we should spend these lives in helping others" (Eph. 2:10, TLB). Chuck Colson was right! We have duties to do as members of the body of Christ through His church.

The next speaker would balance Chuck's viewpoint of "duty" with the reality of heart relationship with the Lord.

Immediately after Chuck's talk, a theologian with a much demurer presentation said, "I don't want to disagree with you, Mr. Colson, but I think it's much more important for us to have the joy of the Lord in our heart than for us to be involved in tasks. It's more important that we be filled with God's Spirit."

The speaker was John Piper, whose books include *The Pleasures of God* and *Desiring God*. In his books he points out the need for the joy of the Lord within our hearts so we enjoy God in our service as well as in our worship.[5] It is easy for us to justify ourselves by our actions, our tasks: giving money, going to the mission field, "doing" in the name of the Lord. But we really cannot have the joy of the Lord in our hearts until we surrender to Him, confess our sins, and ask for His forgiveness, which cleanses our hearts.

Many of Piper's thoughts are aligned with Henry Scougal's treatise, *The Life of God in the Soul of Man*, first published in the late 1600s.[6] Scougal points out that we really cannot ever have God's true joy until we have renounced the desire for the things of the world and have released all our resentments. We cannot have the joy of God until we have surrendered our hearts and lives to Him. We can do all the works in the world, but unless we have His anointing, they do not mean anything.

The Westminster Catechism sums it up this way: "Man's chief end is to glorify God, and to enjoy Him for ever."[7] When we first read that statement, it might seem like very light reading and simplistic theology. It may seem almost too easy to do. But we will come to understand that God does not want just words of praise. He wants us to commit our lives to worshipping Him with a rested heart—one that genuinely feels His presence in our lives. In this way resting becomes a joyful surrender and an abandonment to delight in our Redeemer.

> Therefore, I urge you, brothers and sisters, in view of God's mercy, to offer your bodies as a living sacrifice, holy and pleasing to God—this is your true and proper worship.
>
> —ROMANS 12:1, NIV

When our hearts are resting in Him, we hand over control of our lives; we become living sacrifices. This rested life is the way we worship Him. And when we praise and worship Him with a rested heart, we find true freedom and joy.

> ...so that Christ may dwell in your hearts through faith. And I pray that you, being rooted and established in love,

may have power, together with all the Lord's holy people, to grasp how wide and long and high and deep is the love of Christ, and to know this love that surpasses knowledge—that you may be filled to the measure of all the fullness of God.

—EPHESIANS 3:17–19, NIV

It is that simple and that profound. Exalt, or worship, God. Enjoy Him. Be filled with joy. Our tasks are good, but they must be balanced with religious affections. That balance comes with maturity as a Christian; every "ought to" becomes a "want to." It is just as Jesus said.

I have food to eat that you know nothing about...to do the will of him who sent me and to finish his work.

—JOHN 4:32, 34, NIV

Dear Lord, help me submit to You in love. Help me surrender my heart, mind, and soul to You and rest in the charity that You have given me. Thank You for the joy and felicity that fill my life as I seek to grow in my abandonment to Your promises.

WORSHIP CHANGES US

Praise, love, and enjoyment of God produce in us an everlasting joy as we struggle in a world that is mean and contemptible, that can destroy everything we are and own. All of us have found ourselves encumbered by our worldly lusts. Yet God requires purity and separation from those attitudes, which are constantly seeking to make inroads into our lives.

As we think of God and praise and worship Him, we realize how far short of Him we fall. This is true humility because it results from worshipping God and surrendering ourselves to Him. Humility is not something we decide to acquire. It comes as a result of worshipping Him. As our worship of love becomes all-consuming. It affects every part of our person, and humility becomes ours because we are molded by His Holy Spirit that overflows in us. That humility is essential to enjoying God's fellowship, which is the greatest blessing in our lives.

So by desiring true worship, with faith in His promises above everything else—works, tithing, duties, everything comes into balance. We end up tithing, we end up doing works He ordains for us, and we end up in relationship with Him, exalting *being* before *doing*. In our worship when we exalt Him, we begin to pursue relationship with Him. And as we do, we become more like Him.

> But we all, with unveiled face, beholding as in a mirror the glory of the Lord, are being transformed into the same image from glory to glory, just as by the Spirit of the Lord.
> —2 CORINTHIANS 3:18

When we look in an everyday mirror, we see a reflection of our natural person. But this verse refers to a divine image. Paul wrote of the Word of God as a mirror, reflecting to us the Lord Jesus Christ and His glory. We stand in awe and wonder at such a person, such a Savior, as our Lord Jesus. We behold His glory and want to worship His majesty.

> You make known to me the path of life; you will fill me with joy in your presence, with eternal pleasures at your right hand.
> —PSALM 16:11, NIV

David set before us the reality of fullness of joy in God's presence, joy that comes when we behold God's countenance, when we are caught up in His majesty, and when we surrender ourselves. Being in His presence has to change us because it is so overwhelming.

When we worship His majesty, the Holy Spirit changes us. We are changed into His image from glory to glory. We must learn and relearn every day to put the Lord first, embrace His promises, serve Him, and take Him as our all in all. Our job is simply to adore Him and worship Him. Our greatest desire is that our Maker is pleased. God is infinitely happy in Himself, and nothing is going to shake or unsettle His throne.

In turning back to God, we cannot take offenses personally and internalize them. By internalizing, we actually activate negative change in our biology, our physiology, and our outlook. We begin to think negatively, and it affects who we are. Instead, we must truly look to the Lord with a rested heart and mind to keep us following Him and thinking His thoughts.

One of my friends used to tell me that he needed to pray earnestly a minimum of forty-five minutes each morning. His prayers did not make him perfect, but they brought him closer to God. He had more problems and sins than anybody else would admit, but he was honest enough to admit his failures.

Like him, we have any number of distractions. And like him, prayer is the way back to God when we abandon ourselves and exalt the Lord. That abandonment brings us to a deeper relationship with God, and a more beautiful tranquility and felicity permeate our whole being. We have an afterglow of peace that is overwhelming. When a person comes together with God in worship, he personifies a tranquility that is associated with knowing God, being close to God, worshipping Him in ecstasy, and then having a nature that is changed because of the nearness of God. We become what we pray, and our prayers become the life of God in us. We must be like the Spanish explorer who burned his ships on arrival to America, leaving him without any way of retreat. In our relationship with God, there is no going back on true dedication and abandonment.

The fire of devotion and adoration must always be kept alive by our attitude when we are active in other things. We should be in such a state of worship that life does not become a joyless effort. It becomes a matter of believing in His promises and relaxing in His felicity. Then our lives are transformed from effort and duty to a state of meditation on the glory of God and willing service from the heart.

Only when His majesty truly touches our hearts can His Word fill our whole being. Then those seeds of divine life will flourish and grow because we believe fully in His promises and respond to Him in worship. No longer do we live with worry or want. We surrender our concerns and desires to Him, and we live a life filled with faith and worship. The jewels of His crown enter our eyes, and we see as He sees. It is then that He has truly changed us and we see the glory of God in everything in life and surrender it all to Him.

> But may all who seek you rejoice and be glad in you;
> may those who long for your saving help always say,
> "The LORD is great!"
>
> —PSALM 40:16, NIV

DISCUSSION ❧ QUESTIONS

Describe times in your life when you have worshipped God out of duty and times when you have done so out of love.

....

....

....

....

How does worshipping and exalting God as a result of your love for Him affect your mind and emotions?

....

....

....

....

In what other ways does worshipping God change you?

....

....

....

....

CHAPTER 10

A JOYOUS
LIFE

J OY IS THE natural outpouring of our hearts as we allow God's presence to become the central pillar of our lives. The psalmist declares to God, "You will show me the path of life; in Your presence is fullness of joy; at Your right hand are pleasures forevermore" (Ps. 16:11). How wonderful that sounds! When we embrace God as the central focus of our hearts' desire, we are transformed. We do not look at ourselves and our lives in the same way. We do not worry about events; we do not long for the things of this world; we do not try to find our ultimate happiness in other people or in our work or play. When we turn our entire life over to God, we cannot help but be joyful, for God becomes the source of our joy. We rest securely in His love, confident that He will show us the path of life and fill us with His supernatural joy.

C. S. Lewis wrote about this supernatural transformation in his autobiography. He said that from childhood he found that he was always longing for something that he did not have in his life. Even as a youth, he believed that "something" that was missing was joy. After his conversion to Christ, at the conclusion of his autobiography he asks, "What about my search for joy?" His answer: "After I found God, I didn't think much more about it."[1]

Joy is not found as a result of seeking after joy; it is found only as a result of seeking after Jesus. It is the wonderful emotional expression of our hearts that comes from being centered on Him and not on ourselves. As C. S. Lewis pointed out, joy is a response to the presence of God's love in our souls. People who seek after true godly joy don't look to themselves; they look to God.[2]

There is a story about a professional "memory expert" who appeared on an interview show. In his interview the expert kept calling his interviewer Bob. However, the man's real name was Bill. The interviewer tried correcting the professional a couple of times, but he continued to call his interviewer Bob.

This memory expert, who is supposed to understand how memory works, is like many of us who are supposed to understand the joyful and worshipful heart that is ours as a result of resting in Christ. When we do not show that joy or live in that worshipful attitude, we reflect the incapacity of the memory expert to remember. We think we understand how to have joy but do not remember that it comes only from cultivating a worshipful heart. Our lives reflect His wonderful presence that transforms us only when we spend time worshipping Him. Only in His presence do we receive the fruit and gifts of the Spirit that He has provided for believers, which reflect His divine nature, including joy and peace and His great, loving heart.

Everything in the Bible points out that we must first seek to have a true desire for, and a genuine affection toward, God. When we are focused only on appearances, as the memory expert, we are expressing a religious spirit, which knows the rules but not the heart reality of loving God. When our hearts are surrendered completely to God's will, we experience the heart reality of His love and are filled with joy and felicity.

Dear Lord, may faith in You fill me with Your fruit as You fill my mind with Your Word and presence. Fill

*my soul with joy as You fill my heart with Your love
by the Holy Spirit.*

JOY AND LAUGHTER

The scriptures are filled with admonitions to us to rejoice in
the Lord. The psalmist declared: "Rejoice in the LORD, O ye
righteous: for praise is comely for the upright" (Ps. 33:1, KJV).
Another translation reads: "You are the LORD's people. Obey him
and celebrate! He deserves your praise" (CEV). Holy joy is not an
expression of our own effort to try to build up something within
ourselves. It is an expression of true inner joy that has its source
in our heart relationship with God. And that genuine joy bub-
bles out of us in expressions of love and laughter.

Those who know Chuck Swindoll describe him as a delightful
person who laughs more than anyone else they know. He really
laughs! And it is a genuine expression of joy—he is enjoying himself. He has holy joy! He lives the reality of Paul's exhortation to
believers: "Rejoice in the Lord always. Again I will say, rejoice!"
(Phil. 4:4). All of us should have the joy of God exploding within
us in this way. It should not be uncommon for a believer to burst
out with joy and laughter as we live in the presence of God.

The son of Abraham and Sarah was named Isaac, which
means laughter or he laughs. As an adult, Isaac reopened wells
dug by his father, Abraham, which their enemies the Philistines
had filled up to stop the flow of water. Isaac unstopped those
wells so the water could flow. Similarly genuine, joyful laughter
is an important aspect of freeing ourselves up. Frequently we
become so serious or so burdened by responsibility that we suppress our ability to laugh. This lack of joyful laughter reflects a
lack of genuine fellowship with God due to being caught up in
the cares of life.

But we should live so that we are continually tuned into
the person of Jesus, filled with the spontaneity of emotion, of
laughter, of love, and of caring. Isaac opened up the wells that
had been clogged up by the enemy. Those opened wells gave

freedom to Israel to drink the life-giving water. In the same way, when we live in intimate relationship with the Lord, His joy and laughter release us from negative emotions such as resentment, anger, hate, and bitterness that depress our minds and spirits and fill us with anxiety. The joy of the Lord releases all the stress and anxiety within us and frees us "to glorify God, and to enjoy Him for ever."

Dear God, may my laughter and love come genuinely from You. May my heart be filled with the joy that comes from believing in You.

EXPLOSIONS OF JOY

Finally, brothers and sisters, whatever is true, whatever is noble, whatever is right, whatever is pure, whatever is lovely, whatever is admirable—if anything is excellent or praiseworthy—think about such things. Whatever you have learned or received or heard from me, or seen in me—put it into practice. And the God of peace will be with you.

—PHILIPPIANS 4:8–9, NIV

PAUL TELLS THESE believers first to think correctly so that they can put into practice the genuine life of Christ that he had shown them in his walk with God. Christianity is not just some abstract theory or ideal that we learn in our minds; it is a reality of reflecting the rest of God in our hearts and in our lives through expressions of joy and caring for others. When we truly believe and act out the obedience and direction the Lord calls us to, it is a total life involvement. There is nothing greater than knowing the fullness of that close communion with the living God.

Many people throughout church history have been filled with profound experiences of joy. For example, John Wesley and his friend George Whitefield had been having a rough time working for the Lord. On New Year's Eve in 1738 they bowed their hearts in sincere prayer throughout the night. During this time of prayer they completely abandoned their lives to the Lord. They turned everything over to Him. Then, at about 3:00 a.m. on New Year's Day, a great joy filled both their hearts. They started singing and bursting forth in joy that was almost beyond expression. It seemed their hearts would explode with the intense joy they were experiencing. They were afraid to tell other people what they had experienced for fear others would think they were insane.

Then there was Sarah Edwards, Jonathan Edwards' wife. She went through a period of spiritual dryness in her heart. Then she sought God in a very deep time of prayer. As she waited on God, she received what she described as a "maximum godliness." She developed an enthusiasm and a joy in her life that caused people to wonder at the intensity of her happiness. People thought she was suffering from "distemper and distortion." Jonathan Edwards replied, "If she has distemper, I'd like to have a little of that distemper. And if she's distorted, the whole church should be distorted."[3] He was very proud that his wife had exemplified a deeper walk with God and great godly affection. He observed many who had greater learning and understanding of theology who did not reflect the genuine affections for God that his wife felt. Natural understanding and intellectual knowledge without true affection for God are sterile.

All of us should pursue deeply genuine experiences with God that evoke powerful expressions of love and joy. But there is an appropriate manner in which to do so. Sarah Edwards' words about her own experiences guide us in this important understanding.

> My mind was so deeply impressed with the love of Christ, and a sense of his immediate presence, that I could with difficulty refrain from rising from my seat, and leaping for joy. I continued to enjoy this intense, and lively, and refreshing sense of divine things, accompanied with strong emotions, for nearly an hour, after which, I experienced a delightful calm, and peace and rest in God, until

I retired for the night; and during the night, both waking and sleeping, I had joyful views of divine things, and a complacential rest of soul in God.[4]

When we rest in God and feel privileged to be one with Him, that privilege engenders an appreciation that manifests a joy within our hearts. When our laughter is motivated by Christ Himself, we know we have the true balance that emanates from heavenly joy. May the Spirit of grace enable us as we pray.

Father, I earnestly seek Your presence in my daily life. Fill me with the tranquility that comes from believing in Your promises. Fill me with intense, lively affections as I am ravished with the beauty of the Son of God— my heavenly Bridegroom.

CARING FOR OTHERS

When we are filled with joy, we cannot keep it shut up inside us. It has to express itself and fill all areas of our lives and overflow into our relationships with others. In short, we cannot be truly joyful on the inside yet cranky on the outside. We cannot keep to ourselves the love and joy that fill us when we are in genuine heart communion with God. It pours out of us and onto others. And we are excited to love Him and serve them. Everything we can do that would benefit others makes us rejoice, and we share all their happiness.

When God's rest and joy fill our hearts, we are no longer filled with self-importance. Paul warns against this kind of pride: "If anyone thinks himself to be something, when he is nothing, he deceives himself" (Gal. 6:3). Instead, we allow the instruction of Paul to be reflected through our rested hearts in putting others first.

Do nothing out of selfish ambition or vain conceit. Rather, in humility value others above yourselves, not looking to your own interests but each of you to the interests of the others.

—Philippians 2:3–4, niv

We also find great joy in serving. Psalm 100:2 says to serve the Lord with gladness. The Scottish Metrical Psalms say to serve Him "with mirth." How much easier and more pleasant service is if we do it with mirth and gladness. It is our pleasure, not merely our obligation. And that joy gives us the strength for service—to do the job right.

Remember Mary and Martha? While Mary enjoyed sitting in Jesus' presence, Martha was busy scurrying around to prepare a meal. When we are filled with joy, we are no longer like Martha. We have become like Mary in our hearts, focused on Jesus' love for us and our love for Him. We can still work hard, but our tasks are done joyfully, out of the desire to do well, not just the need to have things done.

In whatever we do, we need to realize that we are aligning ourselves to God and not just trying to work in our own strength. We are working the will of God out of a closeness with God in which we are surrendered to His will.

As we delight in the Lord Jesus as our chief portion in life, we are enabled to be partakers in the happiness of others—their inward endowments and their outward prosperity.

Lord, let me always find my peace, joy, and rest centered in Calvary. May that peace and joy always be within my heart.

DISCUSSION ❧ QUESTIONS

As you've read this book, have you stopped seeking joy in other places and started seeking the rest and joy that is found only in Jesus? Describe how this has affected the anxiety or depression you were experiencing before reading this book.

....

....

....

Since laughter releases you from stress, anger, and worry, how can you be more intentional about making sure you laugh on a daily basis? By enjoying the humor that life's funny situations provoke? By entering into the joy of friends who are experiencing funny situations? By choosing to look on the lighter side of life?

....

....

....

Caring for others can definitely take the focus off your own problems and help lift depression and anxiety. List some ways you will start to care for needs in someone else's life this week.

....

....

....

CHAPTER 11

JOY
AND PEACE

BRAHAM WAS AN old man when his son Isaac was born. God had promised that Abraham would be the father of a great nation. And after a great trial of waiting until that promise seemed impossible to be fulfilled, along came Isaac. Then, after a few years of enjoying this son as the fulfillment of God's promise to give him an heir, God told Abraham to offer Isaac as a burnt offering. Can you imagine? Abraham was being asked to kill his son, his promise received from God, to fulfill all God's promises for the future. But Abraham trusted God. He took Isaac, a knife, and some wood and fire and went up Mount Moriah, exactly as God had told him to do.

Notice his obedient response to this unthinkable command of God. Abraham did not question God; he submitted to God's request and promptly did as God asked. He did not ask others for advice. We do not even know if he informed his wife, Sarah, Isaac's mother. He worked out all the details of the trip and set out. And even though it took three days to reach the place to which God directed him, Abraham still did not doubt God. In faith he kept on going, knowing God would provide the answer to his pain if he obeyed Him. (See Genesis 22.)

Abraham was totally abandoned in faith to God. He was totally surrendered to His will. He was willing to do whatever God asked, knowing God would provide the answer.

> By faith Abraham, when God tested him, offered Isaac as a sacrifice. He who had embraced the promises was about to sacrifice his one and only son, even though God had said to him, "It is through Isaac that your offspring will be reckoned." Abraham reasoned that God could even raise the dead, and so in a manner of speaking he did receive Isaac back from death.
>
> —HEBREWS 11:17–19, NIV

In one of his sermons C. H. Spurgeon noted seven blessings that came to Abraham through his obedience to this trial of his faith.[1] First, the trial was withdrawn, and Isaac was unharmed. Second, Abraham received the highest approval of God for not withholding anything from Him. Third, Abraham saw God in a new light, as One who would be willing to sacrifice His own Son, Jesus, for our sins. Fourth, more of God's nature was revealed. He became known as Jehovah Jireh, the God who provides. Fifth, God confirmed His covenant with Abraham because Abraham proved himself faithful at all costs. Sixth, God reemphasized His promise to Abraham about his offspring. "I will surely bless you and make your descendants as numerous as the stars in the sky and as the sand on the seashore" (Gen. 22:17, NIV). And finally, God gave Abraham a distinct and personal blessing that is perhaps greater than any blessing ever given: blessing promised to all nations of the earth.

> And through your offspring all nations on earth will be blessed, because you have obeyed me.
>
> —GENESIS 22:18, NIV

Imagine Abraham's joy as he came down the mountain with Isaac. His soul must have been filled with exultation, triumph, praise, and glory. God did it! God is faithful! Hallelujah! Abraham must have been overwhelmed and full of joy—the joy of worshipping Jehovah Jireh, the God who provides. Abraham did not have to offer his son. The Lord was his provider.

It is difficult to evaluate the depth of rest and trust in the intimate relationship Abraham had with God. In the same way we must abandon ourselves to God in every circumstance. We must believe in the *Jireh* half of the Lord's name Jehovah Jireh. We must believe that the Lord will provide everything! In His great love God will turn our captivity and cause us to exclaim in joy the wonders of His works in our lives.

> When the LORD brought back the captivity of Zion, we were like those who dream. Then our mouth was filled with laughter, and our tongue with singing. Then they said among the nations, "The LORD has done great things for them." The LORD has done great things for us, and we are glad.
>
> —PSALM 126:1–3

This is the joy of abandoned faith. Abraham went up Mount Moriah filled with faith. He came back down the mountain overwhelmed with joy. We can approach the challenging "mountains" of our own experiences in the same way: climb up with faith in our hearts and go back down filled with joy in God's faithful provision.

Over one hundred years ago C. H. Spurgeon preached a beautiful sermon based on Romans 15:13. I love how Spurgeon tied peace and joy together in that powerful message. He said, "Peace is joy resting, and joy is peace dancing. Joy cries hosanna before the Well-Beloved, but peace leans her head on His bosom."[2] Peace and joy balance beautifully because they balance on Calvary. There is nothing we can do to create that balance. We must be centered on Christ and Calvary, having faith in Him and not in ourselves.

Two godly qualities we see constantly in the lives of early

Christians are their love for Christ and their joy in Christ. These spring from God's love for us and His delight in us. By this inner strength the early Christians gave up all their material things, renounced everything that was dear to them, and faced all kinds of suffering. What happened? Well, the world thought they were crazy. They were imprisoned, tortured, and killed. But that did not stop others from carrying on the mission of sharing the love of Christ to the world. The flame of God's truth kept burning brightly.

These early believers experienced unspeakable joy in their relationship with Christ. They loved God so much that they no longer saw life or responded to hardship with physical eyes. The pearls of God's majesty were transformed in their eyes, and they saw not as the world did but eternal life as God infused them with His life. They saw the unseen—heaven, eternity. They loved Jesus Christ because they saw Him with the eyes of their hearts, and the world saw Him not.

> Though you have not seen him, you love him; and even though you do not see him now, you believe in him and are filled with an inexpressible and glorious joy, for you are receiving the end result of your faith, the salvation of your souls.
>
> —1 PETER 1:8–9, NIV

Like these early believers, we can experience a transforming encounter in God's joy and majesty when we fix our hearts and eyes on Him. We can see as He sees, and our hearts can feel as He feels. We can worship Him and become deeply connected in our hearts to His love and joy. Then we will have true, deeper union and communion with God—in thanksgiving, prayer, service, felicity, rejoicing, and praise.

Jeremiah teaches us one of the indispensable elements of true spiritual joy—the joy that comes from digesting the Word of God. "Your words were found, and I ate them, and Your word was to me the joy and rejoicing of my heart; for I am called by Your name, O LORD God of hosts" (Jer. 15:16). God speaks to us by His Word. He works renewed life in us by the creative power of His Word. He revives our joy as we hear His voice in the Word of God as real as His voice from heaven. The Spirit quickens us, and we experience true communion with the living God.

The practical application we must make is a determination to memorize God's Word. What we do not memorize we will not utilize. We utilize the Word by meditating on it throughout the day, throughout all our daily activities. We utilize it in prayer and in sharing a word in season with others. In many ways the Word "digested" in our hearts causes joy and usefulness to spring up in our lives. Eat the Word as Jeremiah did, and you will find the joy and rejoicing of your heart!

BELIEVING HEARTS CAN TRULY REJOICE

When we truly believe, placing our trust in God, then we will be able to rejoice with joy both inexpressible and full of glory. True faith is receiving God's Word and resting in His redemption. True faith is hearing the Bible not as the word of man, but as the Word of God that has the power to save our souls (Jas. 1:21). That faith is experiencing the reality of Jesus' words.

> My sheep hear My voice, and I know them, and they follow Me.
>
> —JOHN 10:27

True faith is person-to-person dealing with God. Nothing is emptier than a superficial pretense of believing God, not really having faith as the greatest passion of our hearts. True faith includes a humility and repentance that receives Jesus' benediction poured out upon our heads and in our hearts.

> Blessed are the poor in spirit, for theirs is the kingdom of heaven. Blessed are those who mourn, for they shall be comforted.
>
> —MATTHEW 5:3–4

When we believe God's promises from the depth of our hearts, the things that God promises become ours. We are forgiven and can hear Him say the same thing to us as Jesus did to the man let down through the roof at His feet.

> Son, be of good cheer; your sins are forgiven you.
> —MATTHEW 9:2

True faith is an inquiring soul that asks, "Lord, do You care for lepers? Are You willing to cleanse them?" Jesus answers, "I am willing; be cleansed." By faith we possess the promises of God and their fulfillment. Paul wrote the broadest, most encompassing promise of all.

> I will be a Father to you, and you shall be My sons and daughters, says the LORD Almighty.
> —2 CORINTHIANS 6:18

It is reflected in what God said to Abraham.

> I am your shield, your exceedingly great reward.
> —GENESIS 15:1

When we have true faith, we can say with Jeremiah, "The LORD is my portion" (Lam. 3:24). Faith hears God speak to us personally out of His Word by the power of the Holy Spirit, "I will never leave you nor forsake you.... I have loved you with an everlasting love.... Fear not, for I am with you" (Heb. 13:5; Jer. 31:3; Isa. 43:5). Is it any wonder that joy fills the heart and floods the soul of the one who believes God's Word? When we truly drink these promises in and believe them as true for ourselves, then we will rejoice. We are promised a joy that the world cannot give and the world cannot take away.

The essence of living a surrendered, rested life can be summarized in this prayer: *I can't do it without You, Jesus!* We need to die to our selfish perspective of life until we get to that point. We need what A. W. Tozer called a "divine conquest of the soul."[3] God must bring us to see that we have nothing else to trust in except Him. Everything is in the hands of the Son of God. "The Father loves the Son and has placed everything in his hands" (John 3:35, NIV). When we take that posture before God, we can say with David, "Into your hands I commit my spirit," and, "My times are in your hands" (Ps. 31:5, 15, NIV). This is a great morning prayer of surrender and dependence: *I can't do it without You, Jesus!*

Have we been brought to the place in our walk with God where this prayer is the true expression of personal weakness and confidence in the Lord's strength? Is this the way we start our day and return to it often throughout the day? This is the Spirit of God at work in us, reviving us, quickening us, and making us more like Jesus, who depended totally on the heavenly Father. This is the continual work of the kingdom of God in our lives as believers.

> *Lord, sustain our faith and strengthen our joy! May the mystery, the romance, and the joy of totally abandoning ourselves to Your grace enthrall us with You both now and forever.*

DISCUSSION ❧ QUESTIONS

Write down times when God has been faithful to you. Read these when you feel depression or anxiety coming on.

....

....

....

This chapter lists some verses about joy. Write your own list of verses here, and commit them to memory.

....

....

....

Write a prayer of commitment to fully surrender your life into God's care. You can trust Him. Allow His peace that passes all understanding to fill your heart and mind and banish all depression and anxiety as you place your full trust in Him.

....

....

....

....

NOTES

PREFACE

1. *Westminster Shorter Catechism* 1, http://www. westminsterconfession.org/confessional-standards/the-westminster-shorter-catechism.php.

INTRODUCTION

1. Oswald Chambers, *If Ye Shall Ask* (London: Simpkin Marshall, 1937), as stated in Oswald Chambers, *Oswald Chambers: The Best From All His Books*, vol. 1 (Nashville: Oliver Nelson, A Division of Thomas Nelson Publishers, 1987), 250.
2. Henry Scougal, *The Life of God in the Soul of Man* (New York: Cosimo Classics, 2007).
3. Jonathan Edwards, *A Treatise Concerning Religious Affections* (Grand Rapids, MI: Christian Classics Ethereal Library, 1746), https://www.ccel.org/ccel/edwards/affections.html.

CHAPTER 1

1. See, for example, Chris Woolston, "Illness: The Mind-Body Connection," *HealthDay*, updated January 1, 2019, http://blueprint.bluecrossmn.com/topic/depills; "Breast Cancer and Depression," Artemis, accessed February 13, 2019, http://www.hopkinsbreastcenter.org/artemis/200011/feature7.html; Chris Woolston, "Depression and Heart Disease," Blue Cross and Blue Shield of Minnesota, updated March 26, 2003, https://web.archive.org/web/20030415213655/http://blueprint.bluecrossmn.com/topic/depheart.
2. "Mental Health: A Report of the Surgeon General," US Public Health Service, 1999, chapter 1, https://web.archive.org/web/20000303220041/www.surgeongeneral.gov/Library/MentalHealth/chapter1/sec1.html#mind_body.
3. William Collinge, "Mind/Body Medicine—The Dance of Soma and Psyche," *HealthWorld Online*, accessed February

13, 2019, http://www.healthy.net/Health/Article/Mind_Body_Medicine/1949.

4. Andrew Newberg, Eugene D'Aquili, and Vince Rause, *Why God Won't Go Away: Brain Science and the Biology of Belief* (New York: Ballantine Books, 2002), https://books.google.com/books?id=hoCR6B-DjV8C&.

5. Daniel E. Fountain, *God, Medicine, and Miracles* (Wheaton, IL: Harold Shaw Publishers, 1999), 10, https://books.google.com/books?id=_k0fjxQyWv8C&.

6. W. Douglas Brodie, "The Cancer Personality: Its Importance in Healing," W. Douglas Brodie, MD, 2003, https://web.archive.org/web/20030604022618/www.drbrodie.com/cancer-personality.htm.

7. Collinge, "Mind/Body Medicine."

8. "Oswald Chambers Quotes," Goodreads, accessed February 13, 2019, https://www.goodreads.com/quotes/173548-faith-is-deliberate-confidence-in-the-character-of-god-whose.

CHAPTER 2

1. C. H. Spurgeon, "A Round of Delights, No. 1384," Metropolitan Tabernacle Pulpit, November 11, 1877, https://www.spurgeongems.org/vols22-24/chs1384.pdf.

2. C. S. Lewis, *Surprised by Joy: The Shape of My Early Life* (New York: Harcourt Brace, 1955).

3. *Merriam-Webster*, s.v. "relinquish," accessed February 14, 2019, https://www.merriam-webster.com/dictionary/relinquish.

4. John Wesley, *The Journal of John Wesley* (Chicago: Moody Press, 1951), https://www.ccel.org/ccel/wesley/journal.txt.

5. C. S. Lewis, *The Weight of Glory* (Grand Rapids, MI: Zondervan, 2001), 26, https://books.google.com/books?id=WNTT_8NW_qwC&dq.

CHAPTER 3

1. Terry Lindvall, "Joy and Sehnsucht: The Laughter and Longings of C. S. Lewis," *Mars Hill Review* 8 (Summer 1997): 25–38, http://www.leaderu.com/marshill/mhr08/hall1.html.

CHAPTER 4

1. Charles Swindoll, *Laugh Again* (Dallas, TX: Word Books, 1992).

2. Owen Milton, *Christian Missionaries* (Bryntirion, UK: Evangelical Press, 1995), 69.
3. John H. Sammis, "Trust and Obey," 1887, http://www.simusic.com/worship/hymns/.
4. C. H. Spurgeon, *Autobiography* (Edinburgh: Banner of Truth Trust, 1962).
5. Tony Evans, *The Fire That Ignites* (Sisters, OR: Multnomah Publishers, 2003), 10.
6. Richard Baxter, *The Saints' Everlasting Rest* (Lafayette, IN: Sovereign Grace Publishers, 2000), 19, https://books.google.com/books?id=utfTVVO0C-IC&.

CHAPTER 5

1. Earl Palmer, "The Christian Cure for Fatigue," Earl Palmer Ministries, 1996, http://www.earlpalmer.org/wp-content/uploads/2018/02/Fatigue.pdf.
2. Biography at "James Hudson Taylor: Founder of the China Inland Mission," Wholesome Words, accessed February 15, 2019, http://www.wholesomewords.org/missions/biotaylor4.html.

CHAPTER 6

1. Blue Letter Bible, s.v. *"shalowm,"* accessed February 15, 2019, https://www.blueletterbible.org/lang/lexicon/lexicon.cfm?t=kjv&strongs=h7965.
2. *Merriam-Webster*, s.v. "covet," accessed February 15, 2019, https://www.merriam-webster.com/dictionary/covet.

CHAPTER 7

1. Blue Letter Bible, s.v. *"'Iy-kabowd,"* accessed February 15, 2019, https://www.blueletterbible.org/lang/lexicon/lexicon.cfm?t=kjv&strongs=h350.

CHAPTER 9

1. John Piper, *Desiring God: Meditations of a Christian Hedonist* (Colorado Springs, CO: Multnomah Books, 1986), https://books.google.com/books?id=JZiGwLCdE7wC&.
2. Jonathan Edwards, *The Works of Jonathan Edwards* (London: William Ball, 1839).
3. Edwards, *A Treatise Concerning Religious Affections.*
4. Lewis, *Surprised by Joy.*

5. Piper, *Desiring God*; John Piper, *The Pleasures of God: Meditations on God's Delight in Being God* (Sisters, OR: Multnomah Publishers, 1991), https://books.google.com/books?id=YQoJyFlm3A4C&.
6. Scougal, *The Life of God in the Soul of Man*.
7. *Westminster Shorter Catechism* 1.

CHAPTER 10

1. Lewis, *Surprised by Joy*.
2. Lewis, *Surprised by Joy*.
3. Edwards, *The Works of Jonathan Edwards*.
4. Edwards, *The Works of Jonathan Edwards*.

CHAPTER 11

1. Spurgeon, *Autobiography*.
2. Spurgeon, *Autobiography*.
3. A. W. Tozer, *The Divine Conquest* (Old Tappan, NJ: Fleming H. Revell Co., 1950).

ABOUT THE
AUTHOR

J AMES P. GILLS, MD, received his medical degree from Duke University Medical Center in 1959. He served his ophthalmology residency at Wilmer Ophthalmological Institute of Johns Hopkins University from 1962 to 1965. Dr. Gills founded the St. Luke's Cataract and Laser Institute in Tarpon Springs, Florida, and has performed more cataract and lens implant surgeries than any other eye surgeon in the world. Since establishing his Florida practice in 1968, he has been firmly committed to embracing new technology and perfecting the latest cataract surgery techniques. In 1974, he became the first eye surgeon in the United States to dedicate his practice to cataract treatment through the use of intraocular lenses. Dr. Gills has been recognized in Florida and throughout the world for his professional accomplishments and personal commitment to helping others. He has been recognized by the readers of *Cataract & Refractive Surgery Today* as one of the top fifty cataract and refractive opinion leaders.

As a world-renowned ophthalmologist, Dr. Gills has received innumerable medical and educational awards and has been listed in *The Best Doctors in America*. As a clinical professor of ophthalmology at the University of South Florida, he was named one of the best ophthalmologists in America in 1996 by ophthalmic academic leaders nationwide. He has served on the board of directors of the American College of Eye Surgeons, the board of visitors at Duke University Medical Center, and the advisory board of Wilmer Ophthalmological Institute at Johns Hopkins University.

While Dr. Gills has many accomplishments and varied interests, his primary focus is to restore physical vision to patients and to bring spiritual enlightenment through his life. Guided by his strong and enduring faith in Jesus Christ, he seeks to encourage and comfort the patients who come to St. Luke's and to share his faith whenever possible. It was through sharing his insights with patients that he initially began writing on Christian topics. An avid student of the Bible for many years, he has authored numerous books on Christian living, with over nine million copies in print. With the exception of the Bible, Dr. Gills' books are perhaps the most widely requested books in the US prison system. They have been supplied to over two thousand prisons and jails, including every death row facility in the nation. In addition, Dr. Gills has published more than 195 medical articles and has authored or coauthored ten medical reference textbooks. Six of those books were best sellers at the American Academy of Ophthalmology annual meetings.

Did You Enjoy This Book?
We at Love Press would be pleased to hear from you if
God's Rx for Depression and Anxiety
has had an effect on your life or the lives of your loved ones.
Send your letters to:
Love Press
P.O. Box 1608
Tarpon Springs, FL 34688-1608